LOVE YOUR GUT, REVITALIZE YOUR MICROBIOME:

SOOTHE DIGESTIVE ISSUES, BOOST IMMUNITY AND ENERGIZE YOUR LIFE

ELSA RIVERS

CONTENTS

INTRODUCTION

Let's talk about your gut.

Not the six-pack kind or the "gut feeling" kind (though, spoiler alert: they're all connected). I mean the one that keeps you up at night with bloating, discomfort, or an unpredictable schedule. The one that dictates whether you wake up feeling refreshed or sluggish, vibrant or foggy. Your gut does way more than just digest your meals; it's the command center for your health, energy, and emotions.

For years, we've been taught to power through digestive discomfort like it's just part of life, something we deal with rather than heal. But what if I told you that loving your gut is the key to revitalizing your entire body? What if instead of surviving on caffeine, antacids, and stress, you could thrive with energy, clarity, and a sense of well-being you haven't felt in years?

I wrote this book because I've seen firsthand how transformative gut health can be for digestion, immunity, mood, sleep, and overall vitality. Whether you struggle with bloating, IBS, autoimmune issues, or just a general sense of "blah," the good news is this: Your body wants to heal. Your gut is designed to work *for* you, not against you. It just needs the right support.

This isn't another diet book or a quick-fix detox. This is about learning to listen to your body, rebuild a foundation of gut-friendly habits, and create lasting change. Think of it as a guide to reintroducing yourself to your body, one that is capable of resilience, renewal, and deep healing.

We're going to explore the science behind gut health in a way that's easy to digest (pun intended). You'll learn practical, real-life strategies to soothe inflammation, restore balance, and reclaim your energy without perfection, guilt, or overwhelm. Because the goal here isn't just to "fix" your gut. It's to love it. To work *with* it, not against it. To create a relationship with your body that's built on trust and care, rather than frustration and fatigue.

So, if you're ready to stop just getting by and start feeling truly *alive* again, let's get started.

Your gut and your future self will thank you.

On a Personal Note

As I sat in the doctor's office, staring at the lab results in my hands, I couldn't help but feel a mix of confusion and frustration. For years, I had struggled with digestive issues, mood swings, and a weakened immune system, but no one seemed to have the answers I needed. It wasn't until I began to explore the intricate world of gut health that the pieces started to fall into place.

Like many of you, I had no idea just how much our gut influences every aspect of our lives. From the way we digest food to the way we process emotions, the gut plays a central role in our overall health and wellbeing. Yet, despite its importance, gut health remains a mystery to most people, leaving them struggling with a range of issues they can't quite understand.

Recent research has shed light on the gut's incredible complexity, revealing a fascinating ecosystem of microbes that work tirelessly to keep us healthy. These microbes, collectively known as the microbiome, not only help us break down food and absorb nutrients but also communicate with our brain, shaping our moods and influencing our behavior. When this delicate balance is disrupted, whether through poor diet, stress, or other factors, the consequences can be far-reaching.

The purpose of this book is to help you navigate the often-confusing world of gut health and discover the tools you need to transform your well-being from the inside out. Whether you're an adult, young adult or senior, the information and strategies in these pages can help you soothe digestive issues, balance your emotions, boost your immunity, and feel revitalized.

Throughout, we'll explore the latest research on the gut-brain connection, uncovering the ways in which our digestive system and our emotions are intimately linked. We'll also delve into the impact of stress on gut health, offering practical strategies for managing stress and cultivating self-compassion. You'll learn about the power of a plant-based diet and how reducing animal protein is good for your health and emotional balance and beneficial for the environment.

This journey is also about the art of transformation. As we journey through each chapter, you'll discover a roadmap for change, complete with actionable steps and real-life stories of people who have successfully transformed their health by healing their gut. You'll learn how to navigate the social and relationship challenges that can arise when making dietary and lifestyle changes, and you'll find a supportive community of like-minded individuals who are on the same path.

By the end of this book, you'll have a deep understanding of the incredible potential that lies within your gut. You'll know how to nourish your microbiome, soothe your digestive system, and cultivate a sense of emotional balance and resilience. Most importantly, you'll have a vision of what life can look and feel like when your body, mind, and soul are in harmony.

So, if you're ready to embark on a transformational journey to discover the power of gut health and the potential for a vibrant, fulfilling life, then let's dive in together. The path to wellness starts with a single step, and by opening this book, you've already begun.

1

UNDERSTANDING YOUR GUT

On an unremarkable day, as I stood in the kitchen contemplating a simple plate of food, it struck me how complex my relationship with eating had become, fluctuating between moments of indulgence and subsequent guilt. However, the journey of discovering the profound influence of gut health unveiled the true significance of this relationship. The gut, often underestimated, is a marvel of human biology, a bustling metropolis of microorganisms working tirelessly to keep us healthy. This chapter will peel back the layers of this complex world, introducing you to the unsung heroes of digestion and immunity: the microbiome.

1.1 THE MICROBIOME: YOUR INNER ECOSYSTEM

The microbiome is like a bustling city residing within your gut, teeming with a community of bacteria, viruses, fungi, and other microorganisms. These tiny residents play an enormous role in your health, influencing everything from digestion to immune function. In this microbial metropolis, bacteria take center stage, breaking down food and synthesizing essential vitamins like K and B. But the microbiome is not acting alone. Viruses and fungi also contribute, though their roles are less understood. Together, these microorganisms form a symbiotic relationship with the human body, impacting how we metabolize nutrients and fend off pathogens. When this balance is disrupted, the consequences can be far-reaching, affecting not just your gut but your overall health.

Maintaining a balanced microbiome is crucial for optimal health. When the harmony between beneficial and harmful microorganisms is disturbed, a condition known as dysbiosis, various health issues can arise. Dysbiosis has been linked to conditions such as inflammatory bowel disease, obesity, and even mental health disorders. The composition of your microbiome is influenced by your diet and lifestyle. A poor diet, rich in processed foods and low in fiber, can disrupt this balance, allowing harmful bacteria to flourish. On the other hand, a diet rich in diverse plant-based foods supports a healthy microbiome, reinforcing the idea that what you eat directly affects your gut health.

The diversity of your microbiome is a key indicator of its health. A diverse microbiome is like a well-balanced ecosystem, resilient and adaptable to changes. Each species of bacteria plays a unique role, contributing to the overall stability of your gut environment. A varied diet, rich in fruits, vegetables, whole grains, and fermented foods, helps cultivate this diversity, supporting a robust and adaptable microbiome. This diversity not only enhances digestion but also strengthens your immune system, offering protection against a range of diseases.

The functions of the microbiome are as diverse as the organisms that comprise it. One of its primary roles is in digestion, where it aids in breaking down complex carbohydrates into short-chain fatty acids (SCFAs). These SCFAs, such as butyrate, are integral to colon health and have anti-inflammatory properties. The microbiome is also involved in the synthesis of essential vitamins like vitamin K, which is crucial for blood clotting. Furthermore, a healthy microbiome acts as a protective barrier, preventing harmful pathogens from taking hold and causing illness. This intricate dance of microorganisms within your gut underscores the importance of nurturing your microbiome through mindful dietary and lifestyle choices.

Reflection Section: Explore Your Gut Health

Take a moment to consider your current diet and lifestyle. Are you consuming a variety of fruits, vegetables, and fermented foods that support a diverse microbiome? Reflect on any digestive issues you may have experienced and think about how they might relate to the balance of microorganisms in your gut. This awareness is the first step toward making informed choices that promote gut health. Remember, the journey to a healthier gut begins with simple, mindful changes that can have a profound impact on your overall wellbeing.

1.2 GUT-BRAIN AXIS: THE EMOTIONAL LINK

Imagine your gut as a second brain, a complex network communicating directly with your mind. This is the gut-brain axis, a sophisticated system of bidirectional communication that links the gastrointestinal tract and the brain. At the heart of this connection is the vagus nerve, a long meandering nerve that acts as a superhighway for signals traveling between the gut and the brain. This pathway facilitates a continuous dialogue, influencing everything from digestion to mood. Within this system, the gut produces neurotransmitters, the chemical messengers that regulate mood and emotion. Serotonin, often dubbed the "happiness hormone," is predominantly produced in the gut, underscoring its profound influence on emotional wellbeing.

Emotions can wreak havoc on the gut. Stress, anxiety, and mood disorders can dramatically alter gut function, creating a physical response to emotional turbulence. Stress, for example, can change gut motility, leading to symptoms like diarrhea or constipation. Anxiety can exacerbate digestive symptoms, often causing abdominal pain and discomfort. The gut responds to these emotional states with physiological changes, highlighting the intricate dance between mind and body. It's not uncommon to experience a nervous stomach before a big event or feel butterflies when anxious. These sensations are the gut's response to emotional signals, a tangible reminder of the gut-brain connection.

Conversely, the gut exerts a powerful influence on our emotions. A well-functioning gut can foster a stable mood while an imbalanced one may contribute to mood disorders. The production of serotonin in the gut plays a vital role in mood regulation, influencing happiness and anxiety levels. Moreover, the gut microbiota, the community of microorganisms living in the gut, impacts our mental health. Studies have shown that a diverse and balanced microbiota can correlate with lower levels of depression and anxiety. This connection underscores the importance of gut health in maintaining emotional stability and resilience.

Maintaining a healthy gut-brain axis involves proactive strategies. Stress management is crucial, as chronic stress can disrupt the gut-brain connection. Techniques such as mindfulness meditation, yoga, and deep breathing exercises can help manage stress and promote gut health. Dietary choices also play a significant role. Consuming foods rich in omega-3 fatty acids, like salmon and walnuts, can support brain function and reduce inflammation. Fermented foods, such as yogurt and sauerkraut, are beneficial for gut health, promoting a healthy microbiome and enhancing the gut-brain connection.

When considering the gut-brain axis, think of it as an intricate orchestra, where every element must work in harmony to produce a beautiful symphony of health and wellbeing. Like any skilled conductor, you have the power to influence this balance, making choices that nurture both your gut and mind. By understanding and respecting this connection, you can cultivate a life rich in emotional stability and physical vitality. It's a dance of biology and emotion, a testament to the interconnectedness of our bodily systems.

1.3 DEMYSTIFYING GUT FLORA AND ITS FUNCTIONS

Gut flora, often referred to as gut microbiota, constitutes the vast array of microorganisms residing in your digestive tract. These tiny inhabitants are distinct from the broader term "microbiome," which includes all the genetic material of these organisms. While the microbiome is the overarching genetic landscape, gut flora specifically refers to the living organisms themselves. These microbes play a pivotal role in digestion, helping to break down food particles and facilitating nutrient absorption. Imagine them as a bustling workforce, tirelessly processing the nutrients you consume and ensuring they are transformed into forms your body can use efficiently. This process is critical not only for digestion but also for metabolism, as these microorganisms assist in breaking down complex carbohydrates and proteins, providing you with energy and supporting your overall health.

A healthy gut flora acts as a formidable line of defense against various diseases. By maintaining a balanced microbial community, your gut can effectively prevent gastrointestinal disorders such as irritable bowel syndrome and inflammatory bowel disease. Moreover, the influence of gut flora extends beyond the digestive system. Studies have shown that a well-balanced gut microbiota can mitigate the risks of systemic diseases like obesity and diabetes. These conditions are often linked to chronic inflammation and metabolic disturbances, which a healthy gut flora helps regulate. By producing anti-inflammatory compounds and enhancing metabolic efficiency, your gut flora plays a crucial role in disease prevention, acting as a silent guardian of your health.

The role of gut flora in nutrient absorption cannot be overstated. As these microorganisms break down complex carbohydrates, they produce short-chain fatty acids, which serve as an energy source for the cells lining your colon. Additionally, gut flora aids in the absorption of essential minerals, such as calcium and magnesium, which are critical for maintaining strong bones and a healthy nervous system. This process ensures that your body receives the nutrients it needs to function optimally, highlighting the importance of nurturing a healthy microbial community in your gut. By supporting these processes, gut flora contributes significantly to your overall nutritional status and wellbeing.

Despite the significant role gut flora plays in maintaining health, misconceptions abound. One common myth is that taking probiotics alone can ensure a healthy gut flora. While probiotics can introduce beneficial bacteria into your gut, they are not a cure-all. A diverse and balanced diet, rich in fiber and plant-based foods, is essential for supporting a thriving gut flora. Another misconception is that all bacteria in the gut are harmful. In reality, the majority of gut bacteria are beneficial, working symbiotically with your body to enhance health. It's important to recognize that not all bacteria are villains; many are allies that contribute to your wellbeing.

Interactive Element: Gut Health Quiz

Test your knowledge of gut flora with this quick quiz:

1. What is the difference between gut flora and the microbiome?
2. Name two essential functions of gut flora in digestion.
3. How does a healthy gut flora help prevent diseases like obesity and diabetes?
4. What role does gut flora play in nutrient absorption?
5. True or False: Taking probiotics alone can ensure a healthy gut flora.

By understanding the nuances of gut flora, you can make informed decisions about your diet and lifestyle, ultimately supporting a healthier you. As you continue to explore the fascinating world of gut health, remember that these microorganisms are your partners in health, working diligently behind the scenes to keep your body in balance.

1.4 THE SCIENCE OF GUT HEALTH: WHAT YOU NEED TO KNOW

In recent years, the field of gut health has experienced a surge of interest and innovation, driven by projects like the Human Microbiome Project. This ambitious initiative sought to map the diverse microbial populations residing within the human body, particularly in the gut, and understand their impact on health. Through this project, scientists have uncovered the intricate ways in which these microorganisms influence our physical and mental well-being. This research has laid the groundwork for a deeper understanding of how our gut environment interacts with the rest of our body, providing insight into the foundational principles of gut science.

Current research continues to highlight the vital role of the gut in our overall health. Recent studies have established clear links between gut health and chronic diseases such as heart disease, diabetes, and obesity. These conditions often have a connection to inflammation and metabolic dysfunction, both of which are influenced by the state of our gut.

Additionally, emerging therapies are now targeting the microbiome as a means to treat and prevent these diseases. By modulating the gut environment, scientists are exploring new ways to enhance health outcomes and improve quality of life. This shift in focus underscores the gut's pivotal role in disease prevention and management.

A healthy gut environment is crucial for maintaining overall health, acting as a barrier against pathogens and a support system for nutrient absorption. The pH balance within the gut plays a significant role in this process, as it influences the growth of beneficial bacteria and the suppression of harmful ones. A balanced pH creates an environment where good bacteria can thrive, supporting digestion and immune function. Furthermore, the integrity of the gut barrier is vital for preventing harmful substances from entering the bloodstream. When this barrier is compromised, a condition known as "leaky gut" can occur, leading to inflammation and a host of health issues. Maintaining these aspects of gut health is essential for fostering a healthy internal ecosystem.

Based on the latest scientific findings, there are several actionable steps you can take to support gut health. To maintain gut integrity, consider incorporating foods rich in fiber, such as fruits, vegetables, and whole grains, into your diet. These foods nourish beneficial bacteria and help maintain a healthy gut barrier. Additionally, staying hydrated and managing stress are crucial for supporting gut function. Stress can negatively impact the gut environment, so techniques such as meditation, yoga, or deep breathing exercises can be beneficial. Moreover, incorporating fermented foods like yogurt, kefir, and sauerkraut into your meals can introduce beneficial probiotics, promoting a balanced gut microbiome.

As we reach the end of this discussion, it's clear that the gut is a powerful ally in maintaining our health. By understanding the science behind gut health, we can take informed steps to nurture this vital part of our body. The research continues to evolve, but the principles remain the same: support your microbiome, maintain a balanced gut environment, and prioritize your health through mindful dietary and lifestyle choices. By doing so, you can enhance your well-being and set the stage for a healthier, more vibrant life. Embrace the knowledge you've gained, and let it guide you toward better health. Remember, your gut is not only the center of digestion but also a foundation for overall wellness.

2

EMOTIONAL WELLBEING AND YOUR GUT

There was a time when I thought my gut feelings were simply a quirky part of my personality, an inexplicable sense of intuition guiding my choices. It wasn't until I began to explore the science behind these sensations that I realized they were rooted in something far more tangible. Our gut, often referred to as our "second brain," is a powerhouse of emotion and intuition, intricately linked to our mental state. This connection is not just metaphorical; it is grounded in the physical reality of our body's systems.

At the heart of this connection is the intestinal nervous system, a vast network that communicates directly with our brain. This system controls digestion and plays a crucial role in regulating our emotions. It's like having a mini-brain in your belly, constantly sending and receiving signals that influence how you feel. This is why you might feel a knot in your stomach when you're anxious or a flutter of excitement when you're happy. These sensations, often dismissed as mere gut feelings, are actually physiological responses orchestrated by this complex system.

A significant part of this emotional interplay involves neurotransmitters, the chemical messengers that influence mood and behavior. Remarkably, about 95% of the body's serotonin—a neurotransmitter associated with happiness—is produced in the gut. This production is crucial because serotonin helps regulate mood, sleep, and appetite. When serotonin levels are balanced, you feel more content and emotionally stable. Similarly, dopamine, another neurotransmitter produced in the gut, plays a key role in motivation and pleasure. It's the reason you feel a rush of satisfaction after achieving a goal or enjoying a delicious meal. These neurotransmitters underscore the profound impact your gut has on your emotional landscape.

Digestive health significantly affects emotional stability. Conditions like irritable bowel syndrome (IBS) are not just physical ailments; they carry a heavy emotional toll. IBS can lead to anxiety and depression, creating a cycle where emotional distress exacerbates physical symptoms. It's a vicious loop that many find hard to break. Chronic digestive disorders, too, can weigh heavily on mental health, leading to feelings of frustration and helplessness. Understanding this connection can help you take proactive steps to improve both your gut health and emotional well-being.

To enhance your gut feelings and foster emotional balance, consider incorporating gut-friendly foods into your daily meals. Foods rich in fiber, like legumes, nuts, fruits, and colorful vegetables, support a healthy gut microbiome, which in turn can improve your mood and reduce stress. Fermented foods such as yogurt, kimchi, and sauerkraut are excellent sources of probiotics, beneficial bacteria that bolster gut health and emotional resilience. Mindfulness practices, too, can enhance gut awareness, helping you tune into your body's signals and respond with compassion. Techniques such as mindful eating encourage you to savor each bite, improving digestion and fostering a deeper connection with your body.

Reflection Section: Exploring Your Gut-Emotion Connection

Consider keeping a journal to track your gut feelings and emotional responses. Record what you eat and how it makes you feel emotionally and physically. Reflect on how your gut health might be influencing your mood. This practice can offer valuable insights into the intricate dance between your gut and emotions, empowering you to make informed choices that nurture both your body and mind.

This exploration of the gut-emotion connection is just the beginning. As you continue to delve into the relationship between your gut and your mental health, you'll discover a wealth of knowledge and strategies that can transform your wellbeing.

2.1 ANXIETY AND THE GUT: FINDING CALM THROUGH BALANCE

You're familiar with the flutter of nerves before a big event or the gnawing tension during stressful moments. These feelings, often labeled as anxiety, have a surprisingly intimate relationship with your gut health. This connection forms a feedback loop, where anxiety can influence gut function and vice versa. When you're anxious, your body releases stress hormones like cortisol, which can disrupt digestion and alter gut microbiome balance. This disruption, in turn, can exacerbate anxiety, trapping you in a cycle that's hard to break. Understanding this loop is crucial because it reveals how managing your gut health can help alleviate anxiety, providing a pathway to calmer days.

Dietary and lifestyle factors often trigger this cycle. Caffeine and sugar, for instance, are well-known culprits. While they might offer a temporary boost, they can increase anxiety levels by overstimulating your nervous system. Caffeine, found in coffee and energy drinks, can lead to jitters and insomnia, which only heighten anxiety. Sugar, especially in large quantities, can cause spikes and crashes in blood sugar levels, affecting mood and increasing feelings of unease. Sleep deprivation also plays a significant role. Without adequate rest, your body's ability to manage stress weakens, leaving you more vulnerable to anxiety. Ensuring you get enough restorative sleep each night is a simple yet powerful step in calming your mind and gut.

To manage anxiety through gut health, consider your diet. Incorporating foods rich in omega-3 fatty acids, such as salmon, flaxseeds, and walnuts, can be beneficial. Omega-3s are known for their anti-inflammatory properties and their ability to support brain health, which can help stabilize mood and reduce anxiety. Additionally, herbal teas can offer soothing effects. Chamomile and peppermint teas, for example, are renowned for their calming properties. Sipping on these teas can help relax your digestive system and reduce anxiety naturally. These dietary choices act as gentle allies, providing the nutrients your body needs to maintain a balanced emotional state.

Lifestyle changes also play a pivotal role in finding calm. Regular physical activity is a proven stress-buster, with benefits that extend to both mental and gut health. Exercise releases endorphins, the body's natural mood lifters, which can reduce feelings of anxiety. Whether it's a brisk walk, a dance class, or a yoga session, moving your body helps regulate digestion and enhances your overall sense of wellbeing. Yoga, in particular, combines physical activity with relaxation techniques, making it an excellent choice for those seeking to calm both mind and gut. Meditation is another powerful tool. By focusing on the present moment and practicing deep breathing, meditation can help reduce stress and anxiety, promoting a sense of peace and relaxation.

These strategies are not just about managing anxiety; they are about supporting a harmonious relationship between your mind and body. By paying attention to your gut health, you can create a foundation for emotional resilience and a calmer outlook on life.

2.2 MOOD SWINGS AND MICROBIOME: THE HIDDEN CONNECTION

The microbiome, teeming with trillions of bacteria, plays an influential role in how you feel day to day. This vast microbial community within your gut is constantly working behind the scenes, affecting everything from digestion to your emotional state. One of the most intriguing ways it does this is through its impact on hormone regulation. Hormones, those chemical messengers that orchestrate various bodily functions, can be swayed by the balance of bacteria in your gut. When your microbiome is in harmony, these hormones help stabilize mood, ensuring you feel grounded and emotionally balanced. Conversely, when the gut environment is off-kilter, it can lead to hormone imbalances that contribute to mood swings, making you feel emotionally turbulent and unpredictable.

Your microbiome also plays a pivotal role in maintaining neurotransmitter balance, which has a direct impact on your mood. Neurotransmitters such as serotonin and dopamine are crucial for regulating how you feel, and their production can be significantly influenced by the state of your gut. An imbalance in the gut microbiota can lead to fluctuations in these neurotransmitters, which in turn may result in mood instability. This delicate balance highlights the importance of nurturing a healthy gut to promote emotional well-being. When the microbiome is thriving, it supports the production of these mood-regulating chemicals, helping you maintain emotional equilibrium and reducing the likelihood of sudden mood swings.

Dietary choices are a powerful tool in maintaining mood stability. Foods high in sugar and refined carbohydrates might offer a quick energy boost, but they can also cause dramatic spikes and crashes in blood sugar levels. These fluctuations can lead to mood swings, leaving you feeling irritable and emotionally unsettled. On the flip side, whole foods, rich in fiber and nutrients, provide a steady source of energy and help keep your mood stable. Consuming a diet abundant in fruits, vegetables, and whole grains supports your microbiome and, by extension, fosters a more balanced emotional state. These foods not only nourish your body but also promote a sense of well-being, thanks to their positive impact on your gut health.

Inflammation is another key player in the connection between your gut and mood swings. When inflammation occurs in the gut, it can trigger the release of inflammatory cytokines, proteins that communicate with your immune system. These cytokines can affect your brain, potentially leading to mood disturbances. Chronic inflammation has been linked to conditions like depression and anxiety, underscoring the importance of managing inflammation for emotional health. Following an anti-inflammatory diet, rich in foods like fatty fish, leafy greens, and nuts, can help combat inflammation and support a balanced mood. By choosing foods that soothe inflammation, you can create a stable foundation for both gut health and emotional well-being.

Balancing your mood through gut health involves intentional dietary and lifestyle choices. Incorporating probiotic and prebiotic foods into your diet is a practical step toward achieving emotional stability. Probiotics, found in foods like yogurt and kefir, introduce beneficial bacteria into your gut, while prebiotics, present in foods such as bananas and onions, feed the good bacteria already residing there. This combination fosters a thriving microbiome, which in turn supports mood regulation. Additionally, maintaining consistent meal timing can help stabilize blood sugar levels and prevent mood swings. Regular meals provide your body with a steady stream of nutrients, keeping your energy and mood balanced throughout the day.

Incorporating these strategies into your daily routine can significantly impact your emotional well-being. By nurturing your microbiome and making mindful dietary choices, you can support a more stable mood and reduce the frequency of mood swings. It's a holistic approach that acknowledges the profound connection between your gut and emotions, empowering you to take control of your mental health through the choices you make every day.

2.3 EMOTIONAL INTELLIGENCE THROUGH GUT HEALTH

Emotional intelligence might sound like just another buzz-word, but it's a critical element of navigating life's ups and downs. It refers to your ability to understand and manage your emotions and those of others, fostering a sense of empathy and effective communication. You might not realize it, but your gut health can significantly enhance this skill. The gut and brain share a close relationship, and the state of your gut can directly influence your emotional self-awareness. When your gut is in balance, it creates a stable foundation for recognizing and interpreting your feelings accurately, enabling you to respond to situations with clarity and calmness.

A balanced gut doesn't just help you with self-awareness; it also plays a pivotal role in emotional regulation. Think of emotional regulation as the skill that allows you to manage impulses and stress responses. When your gut health is optimal, it supports the production of neurotransmitters that help keep your emotions in check, allowing for better impulse control. This means you're less likely to react impulsively in stressful situations. Moreover, a well-functioning gut helps modulate stress hormones, creating a buffer against the stressors that life throws at you. This buffering effect is crucial for maintaining emotional balance, giving you the resilience needed to handle challenges without feeling overwhelmed.

Beyond personal benefits, emotional intelligence can profoundly impact your relationships and overall quality of life. Heightened emotional intelligence enhances empathy, the ability to understand and share the feelings of others. This empathetic connection can lead to improved relationships because you're more attuned to the emotional needs of those around you. Furthermore, with enhanced emotional clarity, your decision-making capabilities improve. You're able to weigh options more thoughtfully, considering both logical and emotional perspectives. This balanced approach to decision-making can lead to more satisfying outcomes, whether in your personal or professional life.

To nurture emotional intelligence through gut health, consider adopting mindful eating practices. This involves paying close attention to the flavors and textures of your food, as well as how it makes you feel physically and emotionally. By slowing down and savoring each bite, you cultivate a deeper awareness of your body and its signals, enhancing your emotional awareness. Additionally, journaling can be a powerful tool for tracking the connection between your gut and emotions. Regularly jot down what you eat and how you feel afterward. Over time, you'll notice patterns that can inform your dietary choices and emotional responses, offering insights into how to tailor your habits for better emotional balance.

By focusing on your gut health, you can unlock new levels of emotional intelligence, equipping yourself with the tools to navigate life's challenges more effectively. This connection between gut health and emotional intelligence not only enriches your personal experience but also extends to your interactions with the world around you.

As we wrap up this exploration of emotional wellbeing and gut health, consider how these insights can lead to a more harmonious life. By aligning your physical and emotional health, you're setting the stage for a future where both mind and body thrive in unison. With a solid foundation of emotional intelligence, you're better prepared to face the world, equipped with the resilience and empathy needed to foster meaningful connections and a balanced life.

3

NUTRITION FOR A HEALTHY GUT

Growing up, I thought food was just something to fill my stomach, a mundane necessity rather than a powerful tool for health. It wasn't until I started to experience the transformative effects of a plant-based diet that I realized just how impactful our food choices can be. Imagine your gut as a garden, teeming with life, where the right nutrients can cultivate a flourishing ecosystem. This garden thrives on a diverse array of plant-based foods, which not only nourish your body but also create a balanced and vibrant microbiome.

A plant-based diet offers a myriad of benefits for gut health, primarily through its rich fiber content. Fiber acts like a broom, sweeping through the digestive tract and promoting the growth of beneficial bacteria. These bacteria, in turn, play a vital role in maintaining a balanced microbiome, which is crucial for overall health. Plant-based diets are also abundant in phytochemicals—natural compounds found in plants that have been shown to enhance gut health. These compounds possess anti-inflammatory and antioxidant properties, supporting the gut's ability to fend off harmful invaders and reduce inflammation. A systematic review even highlights that such diets can increase beneficial bacteria like Bacteroidetes, contributing to improved gut and overall health (SOURCE 1).

When considering which foods to include in your diet, think of leafy greens like kale and spinach as your new best friends. These greens are packed with fiber and nutrients that support a healthy gut. Legumes, such as lentils and chickpeas, offer another excellent source of fiber and protein. Whole grains like quinoa and oats provide essential nutrients and are known for their positive impact on gut bacteria. Don't forget about nuts and seeds, including almonds and chia seeds, which add healthy fats and fiber to your meals. Together, these foods form the foundation of a plant-based diet, promoting a diverse and balanced microbiome.

Transitioning to a plant-based diet doesn't have to be daunting. Start by incorporating meat-free days into your week. This small change can make a significant impact on your gut health. Gradually introduce plant-based meals for breakfast and lunch, experimenting with different recipes to find what you enjoy. Over time, you'll find that these foods not only benefit your gut but also bring variety and flavor to your diet. The goal is not to restrict but to expand your palate, inviting new tastes and textures into your meals.

For those new to plant-based eating, concerns about protein intake and nutrient deficiencies often arise. Rest assured, there are ample protein sources in plant-based diets. Foods like lentils, chickpeas, tofu, and quinoa are rich in protein and can meet your daily needs. It's also important to ensure you're getting enough essential vitamins, such as B12. While B12 is primarily found in animal products, fortified foods and supplements can bridge this gap. By paying attention to these aspects, you can enjoy the benefits of a plant-based diet without compromising nutrition.

Reflection Section: Plant-Based Diet Exploration

Consider taking a week to explore plant-based eating. Try incorporating at least one plant-based meal a day and keep track of how you feel. Note any changes in your energy levels, digestion, and overall wellbeing. Use this time to experiment with new recipes and flavors, discovering what works best for you. Reflect on the diversity of foods you've introduced into your diet and how they may be impacting your gut health. This exercise can provide valuable insights as you continue your journey toward a healthier, more balanced lifestyle.

3.1 FOODS THAT HEAL: PROBIOTICS AND PREBIOTICS

Picture your gut as a bustling, microscopic city, where probiotics and prebiotics are the key players keeping everything running smoothly. Probiotics, often called "good" bacteria, are live microorganisms that bring a host of benefits to your digestive system. They help maintain a healthy balance of gut bacteria, which is crucial for digestion and immune function. When your gut is populated with these beneficial bacteria, it can fend off harmful invaders more effectively, keeping you healthier and less prone to infections. On the other hand, prebiotics are the unsung heroes that feed these good bacteria. They are non-digestible fibers found in certain foods that travel to the colon, where they serve as nourishment for probiotics. This dynamic duo works in harmony to support a thriving gut environment, enhancing your overall wellbeing.

Incorporating probiotic-rich foods into your diet is a delicious way to boost your gut health. Yogurt and kefir are classic examples, both packed with live cultures that replenish your gut flora. These creamy, tangy foods can be enjoyed on their own or added to smoothies for a tasty, gut-friendly treat. Fermented vegetables, such as sauerkraut and kimchi, offer another flavorful avenue for probiotics. These foods not only add zest to your meals but also introduce a variety of beneficial bacteria to your gut. Kombucha, a fizzy and refreshing probiotic beverage, has gained popularity for its gut-boosting properties. Made from fermented tea, kombucha is a great alternative to sugary sodas, providing a natural and healthful effervescence.

Prebiotics, while less glamorous, are equally important in maintaining gut health. Garlic and onions, staples in many kitchens, are rich in prebiotic fibers. These aromatic ingredients can easily be incorporated into a wide range of dishes, acting as a flavorful base for soups, stews, and sauces. Bananas are another excellent prebiotic source, offering a sweet and convenient snack that supports gut health. Asparagus, often celebrated for its nutrient content, also serves as a great prebiotic food. Chicory root and Jerusalem artichokes round out the list, though they might not be as common in your pantry. These foods can be roasted or added to salads and are worth trying for their prebiotic benefits.

Incorporating probiotics and prebiotics into your daily meals doesn't have to be complicated. Start your day with a smoothie made with probiotic-rich yogurt, blending in fruits and a handful of spinach for an extra nutrient boost. Use garlic and onions as foundational ingredients in your cooking, enhancing both flavor and gut health. When preparing salads, consider adding prebiotic-rich vegetables like asparagus or Jerusalem artichokes. These simple adjustments can make a significant difference, ensuring that your gut receives the nourishment it needs to thrive. With a bit of creativity, these foods can become a seamless part of your everyday diet, supporting a healthy and balanced microbiome.

3.2 AVOIDING DIETARY PITFALLS: WHAT TO SKIP

Navigating the modern food landscape can feel like walking through a minefield, especially when it comes to protecting your gut health. Many common dietary habits can quietly sabotage your microbiome, leading to a host of health issues. High sugar consumption is one of the primary culprits. When you consume excessive amounts of sugar, it can lead to dysbiosis, a condition where the balance of gut bacteria tilts unfavorably. Harmful bacteria thrive on sugar, crowding out the beneficial ones that keep your gut healthy. Over time, this imbalance can contribute to digestive discomfort, weight gain, and even mood swings. Processed foods, often laden with hidden sugars and additives, further exacerbate this issue. These convenient but nutritionally void foods can strip your gut of its natural defenses, leaving it vulnerable to inflammation and disease.

Artificial additives present another hidden threat to gut health. While they may enhance flavor or extend shelf life, preservatives and artificial sweeteners can disrupt the delicate ecosystem of your gut. Aspartame, a common artificial sweetener, has been shown to alter gut bacteria, potentially leading to digestive issues and metabolic changes. Similarly, preservatives, which are designed to kill bacteria, don't discriminate between harmful and beneficial microbes. This can lead to a reduction in the diversity of your microbiome, weakening its ability to protect against pathogens and maintain overall health. The impact of these additives is subtle but significant, often manifesting as bloating, irregular bowel movements, or a general feeling of malaise.

Excessive alcohol and caffeine consumption can also wreak havoc on your gut. While a glass of wine or a cup of coffee can be enjoyed in moderation, overindulgence can harm gut function. Alcohol can damage the gut lining, leading to increased intestinal permeability, often referred to as "leaky gut." This condition allows toxins and undigested food particles to enter the bloodstream, triggering inflammation and a cascade of health problems. Caffeine, on the other hand, can irritate the digestive system, especially for those who are sensitive. It can increase stomach acid production, leading to discomfort and exacerbating conditions like acid reflux or gastritis. Moderation is key, and being mindful of your intake can help maintain a healthy gut environment.

Making healthier dietary choices involves a proactive approach. Start by scrutinizing food labels to identify hidden sugars and additives. Many products marketed as "healthy" or "low-fat" might be loaded with sugars and chemicals to improve taste. Opt for whole foods instead of processed snacks. Whole foods, such as fruits, vegetables, nuts, and seeds, provide natural nutrients and fiber that support gut health. They don't contain the additives and preservatives that can disrupt your microbiome. By choosing whole foods, you're not only nourishing your body but also supporting a diverse and balanced gut environment.

A practical strategy to reduce sugar and additive intake is to prepare meals at home. Cooking from scratch allows you to control what goes into your food, ensuring that you're not inadvertently consuming harmful substances. Experiment with herbs and spices to enhance flavor without relying on sugar or artificial ingredients. Additionally, when dining out, be aware of menu items that may contain hidden additives. Don't hesitate to ask for modifications or ingredient lists. Being informed and proactive in your food choices can significantly impact your gut health, paving the way for better digestion, mood stability, and overall wellness.

3.3 SUSTAINABLE EATING FOR A HEALTHIER GUT

In recent years, there has been a growing awareness of the connection between our dietary choices and the health of our planet. Sustainable eating practices not only benefit the environment but also play a crucial role in enhancing gut health. When you choose to eat sustainably, you're essentially making decisions that positively impact both your body and the world around you. One of the key aspects of sustainable eating is minimizing the environmental impact of our food consumption. Plant-based diets, for instance, are known to have a lower carbon footprint compared to diets rich in animal products. By reducing the consumption of meat and dairy, you not only decrease greenhouse gas emissions but also support a diverse and balanced gut microbiome.

Organic foods are another essential component of sustainable eating. They are grown without the use of synthetic pesticides and fertilizers, which can harm both the environment and your gut. Organic farming practices support healthier soil and ecosystems, which in turn promote a richer microbial diversity in the food we consume. This diversity is reflected in your gut microbiome, enhancing its ability to digest food, fend off pathogens, and support overall health. By choosing organic produce, you're not only reducing your exposure to harmful chemicals but also nurturing your gut flora.

When it comes to sustainable food choices, there's a growing emphasis on seasonal and local produce. These foods are often fresher and require less transportation, reducing their carbon footprint. Seasonal produce is harvested at its peak, offering superior taste and higher nutrient content. By supporting local farmers and markets, you contribute to a more sustainable food system and gain access to a variety of fresh, gut-friendly ingredients. Additionally, mindful consumption plays a critical role in reducing food waste. Planning meals and properly storing leftovers can help minimize waste, ensuring that every part of your food finds a purpose.

Reducing animal products in your diet offers both health and environmental benefits. Lowering your intake of saturated fats, commonly found in red meat and dairy, can improve cardiovascular health and reduce inflammation. From an environmental perspective, livestock farming is a major contributor to greenhouse gas emissions, water pollution, and deforestation. By choosing plant-based alternatives, you reduce your carbon footprint and support a more sustainable agricultural system. This shift doesn't require eliminating animal products entirely but encourages moderation and balance for a healthier lifestyle.

Transitioning to sustainable eating practices might seem challenging, but it can be achieved through simple, gradual steps. Begin by planning meals based on seasonal availability. This approach not only ensures fresher produce but also introduces variety into your diet, keeping your meals exciting and diverse. Explore local farmers' markets to discover fresh ingredients and support your community. Engaging with local producers can also provide insights into sustainable farming practices and inspire you to make informed choices.

As you embrace sustainable eating, remember that small changes can lead to significant impacts. By aligning your dietary habits with the values of sustainability, you're contributing to a healthier planet and a more resilient gut.

This chapter has highlighted the profound connection between sustainable eating and gut health, showing how mindful choices can create a ripple effect of benefits. In the next chapter, we will explore how boosting your immunity through gut health can be a game-changer for overall wellbeing.

4

BOOSTING IMMUNITY THROUGH GUT HEALTH

Imagine your gut as a bustling fortress, its walls lined with vigilant guards ready to fend off invaders. This fortress is a crucial part of your immune system, a dynamic network that tirelessly defends against pathogens. At the heart of this defense is the gut-associated lymphoid tissue (GALT), a powerhouse of immune activity nestled within your digestive tract. GALT forms a vital component of the immune system, accounting for about 70% of its weight. It operates as a training ground for immune cells, teaching them to distinguish between harmful invaders and harmless substances. This system is essential because the gut's mucosal surface is vast and permeable, making it a prime target for pathogens. By training immune cells, GALT ensures that your body can mount a robust defense against potential threats.

The gut lining acts as a formidable barrier, akin to a moat protecting a castle. It regulates the passage of nutrients while preventing toxins and pathogens from slipping through. When this barrier functions optimally, it keeps harmful substances at bay, maintaining the integrity of your internal environment. However, when compromised, it can lead to increased intestinal permeability, often referred to as "leaky gut." This condition allows unwanted particles to enter the bloodstream, triggering inflammation and potentially leading to autoimmune conditions. Maintaining a healthy gut lining is crucial for a resilient immune system, as it forms the first line of defense against invaders.

Within this intricate system, beneficial bacteria play a pivotal role in modulating immune responses. These bacteria, part of the gut microbiota, produce short-chain fatty acids (SCFAs) through the fermentation of dietary fibers. SCFAs serve as communication signals, influencing both innate and adaptive immunity. They enhance the activity of immune cells, such as macrophages and natural killer cells, which target and destroy pathogens. Additionally, SCFAs help regulate inflammation by inhibiting the production of pro-inflammatory cytokines. This dual role underscores the importance of nurturing a diverse and balanced microbiota, as it directly impacts your body's ability to fend off infections.

When the gut is compromised, the consequences can be far-reaching. A weakened gut can lead to increased susceptibility to infections, as the body's defenses are unable to mount an effective response. Chronic inflammation, often a result of a disrupted gut microbiota, can further exacerbate immune dysfunction, paving the way for autoimmune conditions. These conditions arise when the immune system mistakenly attacks healthy cells, perceiving them as threats. A healthy gut is central to preventing these issues, as it supports immune homeostasis and reduces the risk of chronic inflammation.

To support the gut-immune connection, consider incorporating fiber-rich foods into your diet. Foods like fruits, vegetables, and whole grains provide the essential fibers needed for beneficial bacteria to thrive. These fibers serve as fuel for the production of SCFAs, promoting a balanced microbiota and enhancing immune function. Maintaining hydration is equally important, as water supports optimal gut function and helps flush out toxins. Drinking adequate water ensures that your digestive system operates smoothly, facilitating the absorption of nutrients and the elimination of waste.

Reflection Section: Assess Your Gut-Immune Health

Take a moment to evaluate your current diet and lifestyle. Are you consuming enough fiber-rich foods to support a healthy gut microbiota? Consider keeping a food diary to track your fiber intake and its impact on your overall wellbeing. Reflect on your hydration habits as well. Are you drinking enough water to support your gut's functions? This reflection can provide insights into areas for improvement, guiding you toward a healthier gut and a stronger immune system.

4.1 NATURAL IMMUNITY BOOSTERS: A GUT-CENTRIC APPROACH

Imagine your kitchen as a pharmacy of natural remedies, where the right foods not only nourish the body but also fortify your immune system. Citrus fruits, with their vibrant colors and refreshing flavors, are a prime example of this dual benefit. Packed with vitamin C, they not only support immune function by boosting white blood cell production but also enhance gut health by acting as prebiotics. When you enjoy a juicy orange or a tart grapefruit, you're not just satisfying your taste buds—you're feeding your gut micro-biota, encouraging a thriving community of beneficial bacteria. The same can be said for ginger, a humble root with powerful anti-inflammatory properties. Known for its ability to soothe digestive discomfort, ginger also supports immune function by reducing inflammation, a key factor in both gut and immune health. Incorporating these foods into your diet can create a strong foundation for a resilient immune system.

Herbs and spices, often relegated to the role of flavor enhancers, are actually potent allies in the quest for better health. Take turmeric, for instance, with its active compound curcumin. This bright yellow spice is renowned for its anti-inflammatory and antioxidant properties, making it a valuable addition to any diet. Curcumin has been shown to modulate immune responses, supporting the body's ability to fight off infections while maintaining gut health. Echinacea, another powerful herb, is often associated with immune support. It works by enhancing the activity of immune cells, fortifying the body's defenses against pathogens. Meanwhile, garlic, with its pungent aroma, boasts antibacterial and antiviral effects. Its compounds can help maintain a balanced gut microbiome by inhibiting the growth of undesirable bacteria and viruses, offering a protective shield for your entire system. These herbs and spices, when used regularly, can transform ordinary meals into nourishing, immunity-boosting feasts.

Fermented foods are like the secret weapon in your dietary arsenal, quietly working to enhance both gut and immune health. Miso and tempeh, staples in many Asian cuisines, are excellent sources of probiotics, the beneficial bacteria that support a balanced gut microbiota. By regularly consuming these foods, you introduce a diverse array of probiotic strains into your system, promoting digestive health and bolstering immune function. Kefir, a fermented dairy product, is another powerful probiotic food. It's rich in a variety of beneficial bacteria and yeasts, which can help maintain gut balance and support immune health. Including fermented foods in your diet can lead to increased microbial diversity, a key factor in a resilient immune system, as noted in studies showing their impact on reducing inflammation and enhancing gut health.

Bringing these immunity-boosting foods into your daily routine can be both simple and delicious. Consider starting your day with a cup of ginger-turmeric tea. Simply steep slices of fresh ginger and turmeric in hot water, adding a splash of lemon juice and a drizzle of honey for added flavor. This soothing beverage not only warms you from the inside out but also provides a gentle boost to your immune system. For lunch or dinner, try a fermented vegetable stir-fry. Sauté a mix of your favorite vegetables—such as bell peppers, broccoli, and carrots—in a bit of olive oil. Add a scoop of kimchi or sauerkraut for a tangy kick and a dose of probiotics. Serve this colorful medley over a bed of brown rice or quinoa for a meal that's as nutritious as it is satisfying.

4.2 ILLNESS PREVENTION: GUT STRATEGIES FOR A RESILIENT BODY

In the quest for robust health, it's essential to consider the simple yet effective routines that can bolster your immune defenses. Regular handwashing stands out as a fundamental practice. By washing your hands frequently, you reduce the risk of transferring harmful pathogens to your gut. This simple habit can prevent a myriad of infections, acting as a first line of defense in your daily life. Another key strategy involves being mindful of antibiotic use. While antibiotics are powerful tools against bacterial infections, their overuse can disrupt the delicate balance of your gut microbiota, leaving your immune system vulnerable. It's crucial to use antibiotics only when necessary and as prescribed by a healthcare professional.

Stress management is another critical component of maintaining a strong immune system. Chronic stress can wreak havoc on your gut health and, by extension, your immunity. Stress can increase the permeability of your gut lining, leading to what is often termed "leaky gut." This condition allows toxins and bacteria to enter the bloodstream, triggering inflammation and weakening your immune response. Incorporating stress reduction techniques into your daily routine can make a significant difference. Deep breathing exercises, for example, can help lower stress levels, promoting relaxation and balance in your body. Other practices, like yoga or meditation, can also be effective, helping you manage stress and protect your gut and immune health.

Adequate sleep is non-negotiable for a healthy immune system. During sleep, your body undergoes critical repair processes, including the maintenance of your gut microbiome. Sleep deprivation can disrupt this balance, weakening your immune defenses and leaving you more susceptible to illness. To improve sleep quality, establish a regular sleep schedule, going to bed and waking up at the same time each day. Creating a calming bedtime routine, such as reading or listening to soothing music, can also signal to your body that it's time to wind down. Ensuring your sleeping environment is dark, quiet, and cool can facilitate more restful sleep, supporting both gut and immune health.

To maintain a resilient immune system, consistency in your daily habits is key. Eating meals at regular intervals can support digestive health by optimizing gut function and ensuring steady energy levels throughout the day. This consistency can prevent digestive disturbances and promote a balanced microbiome. Additionally, incorporating mindfulness practices into your routine can enhance overall wellbeing. Simple mindfulness exercises, such as focusing on your breathing or taking a few moments to appreciate your surroundings, can help reduce stress and promote mental clarity. These practices not only support your mental health but also create a harmonious environment for your gut, fostering resilience and vitality in your immune system.

4.3 LONG-TERM HEALTH: BUILDING IMMUNE RESILIENCE

Imagine a world where your immune system is not just reactive but resilient, adapting to threats with the precision of a seasoned strategist. This concept of immune resilience is about more than just fighting off today's cold or flu—it's about building a foundation for lifelong health. Your immune system is inherently adaptive, designed to learn and respond to new challenges over time. This adaptability is largely supported by the diversity of your gut microbiota. A diverse microbiome equips your immune system with a broader range of tools to recognize and neutralize pathogens, promoting a state of readiness and balance.

Maintaining a healthy gut is akin to investing in a lifelong insurance policy for your immunity. A robust gut can significantly decrease the risk of chronic diseases such as heart disease, diabetes, and even certain cancers. By supporting a balanced microbiome, you're effectively reducing inflammation, a key driver of many chronic conditions. A healthy gut also enhances recovery from illnesses. When your gut is in good shape, it can more efficiently absorb nutrients and support the body's natural repair processes, helping you bounce back faster when sickness does strike. This not only improves your quality of life but also ensures that your immune system is always at its best, ready to defend against new threats.

To build and maintain immune resilience, consider a proactive approach that includes periodic dietary assessments. Regularly evaluate your diet to ensure it provides the necessary nutrients to support both gut and immune health. This might involve keeping a food diary or consulting with a nutritionist to make informed adjustments. Pair this with regular physical activity, which is known to boost immune function and maintain gut health. Exercise stimulates the production of anti-inflammatory cytokines and enhances circulation, ensuring that immune cells are distributed effectively throughout the body. Whether it's a daily walk, a yoga session, or a run, finding an activity you enjoy will make it easier to stay consistent.

Taking control of your health begins with setting clear, achievable goals. Focus on specific aspects of your gut and immune health that you want to improve, and set realistic targets. Perhaps you want to increase your daily fiber intake or commit to a weekly exercise routine. Whatever your goals, write them down and track your progress. This practice not only holds you accountable but also allows you to celebrate small victories along the way. Creating a supportive environment is equally important. Surround yourself with resources and people who encourage healthy living. This might mean stocking your kitchen with nutritious foods, joining a fitness group, or engaging with online communities focused on wellness. The support you build around yourself can be a powerful motivator, helping you maintain a healthful lifestyle over the long term.

By nurturing your gut, you lay the groundwork for a resilient immune system, capable of withstanding the tests of time. This chapter has highlighted the importance of immune resilience and the role of gut health in achieving it. As you continue to explore the connections between your gut and overall health, you'll discover even more ways to foster a balanced, vibrant life.

5

PRACTICAL LIFESTYLE CHANGES

S tress is a part of life, just like the sun rising each morning. Whether you're racing against deadlines or navigating the maze of relationships, stress finds a way to sneak into your day. I remember a time when stress was my constant companion, casting shadows on my gut health. It wasn't the deadlines or personal challenges themselves, but how they seemed to tie my stomach in knots. This chapter dives into understanding how stress impacts your gut and how you can create a haven of calm amidst the chaos.

Chronic stress doesn't just live in your mind; it takes up residence in your body, particularly in your gut. When you're stressed, your body releases cortisol, a hormone designed to help you handle situations that require a quick response. While cortisol is useful in short bursts, chronic stress leads to elevated cortisol levels that can throw your digestive system off balance. This hormone can slow down digestion, leading to issues like bloating and discomfort. It can also alter gut motility, the way your intestines contract to move food along. This can result in constipation or, conversely, diarrhea—a reminder that your gut is listening to your emotions.

Work and personal life are common culprits when it comes to stress that impacts the gut. The pressure of meeting work deadlines can feel like carrying a weight on your shoulders, often manifesting as tightness in your stomach. Similarly, emotional stress from personal relationships, whether it's a disagreement with a friend or family tension, can trigger a gut reaction. These stressors aren't just fleeting moments; they can linger, affecting your gut health over time. It's important to recognize these triggers and understand how they may be impacting your digestion and overall wellbeing.

Fortunately, there are ways to manage stress and protect your gut health. Progressive muscle relaxation is a technique that involves tensing and then relaxing different muscle groups in your body. This practice can help reduce physical tension and bring a sense of calm to your mind. Breathing exercises offer immediate relief. By focusing on your breath and taking slow, deep breaths, you can calm your nervous system and reduce stress levels. Regular breaks throughout your day are also essential. They give your mind a chance to reset and can improve your productivity. Implementing time management strategies helps ensure these breaks are part of your routine, reducing stress and protecting your gut.

Creating a stress-reducing environment at home or work is another powerful tool. Consider incorporating plants and natural elements into your living space. Plants not only purify the air but also create a sense of tranquility. They act as a gentle reminder of nature's calm amidst the hustle of daily life. Setting boundaries for work-life balance is equally important. Make sure you allocate time for relaxation and leisure, free from the demands of work. This balance is vital for maintaining your mental health and, by extension, your gut health.

Reflection Section: Your Stress Management Toolkit

Take a moment to reflect on your current stress levels and how they might be affecting your gut health. What are your primary sources of stress? Consider jotting down a list of stressors. Next, choose one stress-reduction technique from this chapter to incorporate into your daily routine. Whether it's a breathing exercise or adding a plant to your space, commit to trying it for a week. Note any changes in your stress levels or gut health. This practice can help you build a personal toolkit for managing stress, paving the way for a healthier, more balanced life.

5.1 SLEEP AND GUT HEALTH: THE RESTORATIVE LINK

Picture this: you're lying in bed, tossing and turning, struggling to find that elusive sleep. What you might not realize is that your gut is also yearning for rest. Sleep does more than recharge your mind; it plays a pivotal role in gut repair and regeneration. During those precious hours of slumber, your body shifts into a state of healing, working diligently to repair the gut lining and balance the microbiome. This restorative process is crucial because a healthy gut supports everything from nutrient absorption to immune function. However, when sleep is disrupted, this critical repair work stalls, leaving your gut vulnerable to imbalances and inefficiencies.

Sleep deprivation has a tangible impact on gut flora diversity. Just as a diverse garden thrives, a gut teeming with a variety of bacteria is a hallmark of health. But lack of sleep can alter this diversity, tipping the scales toward less beneficial microbes. This imbalance can lead to digestive issues and a weakened immune system, highlighting the importance of quality sleep for maintaining a robust gut. Moreover, insufficient sleep can increase inflammation, a silent disruptor that quietly undermines gut health. Inflammation can lead to discomfort and even exacerbate conditions like irritable bowel syndrome, making it clear that sleep is an integral part of the gut-health equation.

Poor sleep doesn't just stay confined to your bed; it ripples through your entire body, affecting your gut and beyond. When you're sleep-deprived, the communication between your gut and brain can falter. This disruption can lead to a vicious cycle where your gut feels out of sync, affecting everything from mood to digestion. As the gut-brain axis misfires, you might notice increased cravings for unhealthy foods, which can further upset your gut balance. This cycle underscores the interconnectedness of your body's systems and the critical role sleep plays in maintaining harmony.

To support both your sleep and gut health, consider establishing a regular sleep schedule. Going to bed and waking up at the same time each day helps regulate your body's internal clock, making it easier to fall asleep and wake up refreshed. Creating a bedtime routine that promotes relaxation can also enhance your sleep quality. Simple practices like reading a book, taking a warm bath, or listening to calming music signal to your body that it's time to wind down. These rituals not only prepare your mind for rest but also encourage your gut to enter its restorative state.

Transforming your sleeping environment can make a world of difference in the quality of your sleep. Start by reducing noise and light pollution in your bedroom. Consider investing in blackout curtains to block out unwanted light and using a white noise machine to mask disruptive sounds. These changes create a serene atmosphere that invites restful sleep. Your mattress and pillows also play a crucial role in sleep quality. Choose options that provide the right balance of support and comfort, ensuring that you wake up without stiffness or pain. A comfortable bed is more than a luxury; it's a foundation for good sleep and, by extension, a healthy gut.

5.2 EXERCISE AND THE MICROBIOME: MOVING TOWARDS BALANCE

Physical activity is often seen as a way to keep the body fit, but its benefits extend far into the realm of gut health. Exercise is like a natural fertilizer for your microbiome, promoting growth and diversity among the gut's microbial residents. When you engage in regular physical activity, you encourage an increase in gut microbial diversity. This diversity is a hallmark of robust gut health, supporting everything from digestion to immune function. The more varied your gut microbes, the better equipped your body is to digest food and fend off pathogens. Exercise also enhances gut motility, which is the process that moves food through your digestive tract. Improved motility ensures that food is digested efficiently, reducing bloating and discomfort. It's a reminder that your body thrives on movement, inside and out.

Certain types of exercise are particularly beneficial for gut health. Moderate aerobic activities, such as walking and cycling, are excellent choices. They gently boost heart rate and circulation, which in turn supports gut function. Walking is accessible and can be easily integrated into daily life, making it a versatile option for anyone looking to support their gut. Cycling, whether outdoors or on a stationary bike, offers a similar benefit with the added bonus of strengthening the lower body. Strength training also plays a role in overall body health and subsequently, gut health. By building muscle, you enhance metabolism and support the body's ability to process nutrients effectively. This type of exercise doesn't need to be intense; simple bodyweight exercises or using resistance bands can yield significant benefits for your gut.

Incorporating exercise into your daily routine doesn't have to be a chore. Consider the idea of walking meetings if your work environment allows. Instead of sitting in a conference room, take the discussions outside or through the corridors. This approach not only gets you moving but also stimulates creative thinking. Short, high-intensity interval training (HIIT) sessions are another way to integrate exercise into a busy schedule. These workouts are efficient and can be done in as little as 15-20 minutes, offering a full-body workout that promotes cardiovascular and gut health. The key is to find activities that you enjoy and can maintain consistently.

While exercise is crucial, it's important to approach it with balance. Over-exertion can lead to burnout and even harm your gut health by increasing stress levels. Listen to your body's signals and recognize when it needs rest. This intuitive approach helps prevent injury and supports long-term wellness. Balancing different types of physical activities is also crucial. Incorporating a mix of aerobic, strength, and flexibility exercises ensures that your body receives comprehensive benefits. This variety not only keeps workouts interesting but also addresses different aspects of health, from cardiovascular fitness to muscle strength and flexibility.

Exercise is a powerful tool for supporting gut health, and its benefits are within reach for everyone. By understanding how different forms of activity impact your body, you can make informed choices that promote a healthy microbiome and overall wellbeing.

5.3 MINDFULNESS PRACTICES FOR GUT WELLBEING

Mindfulness isn't just a trendy buzzword; it's a powerful practice that can bring harmony to your body and mind. At its core, mindfulness is about being fully present and engaged in the moment, without judgment. This practice has a profound impact on gut health, offering a pathway to reduce stress and promote emotional balance. When you engage in mindfulness, you activate the parasympathetic nervous system, which calms the body and aids digestion. The gut-brain connection thrives when you're mindful, as you're more attuned to your body's signals and needs. This awareness can help you make better choices that support both your mental and physical health.

Integrating mindfulness into daily life can transform ordinary activities into opportunities for growth and healing. Mindful eating is a technique that enhances digestion by encouraging you to savor each bite and listen to your body's hunger cues. By slowing down and truly tasting your food, you allow your digestive system to work more efficiently. Meditation is another powerful tool in the mindfulness arsenal. Regular practice can calm the digestive system by reducing stress and promoting a sense of inner peace. Even short, daily sessions can help you feel more centered and less reactive to life's challenges. Body scan exercises, where you mentally check in with different parts of your body, increase awareness and help you recognize areas of tension or discomfort. This practice can guide you to make adjustments that improve your overall wellbeing.

To make mindfulness a regular part of your routine, start by setting aside time each day for meditation or reflection. Even just five minutes can make a difference. Consider using mindfulness apps for guided practices, which can provide structure and inspiration. These tools are accessible and can be tailored to fit your schedule, helping you develop a consistent practice. The key is to approach mindfulness with an open mind and a willingness to explore its benefits. As you cultivate this practice, you'll likely notice improvements in both your mental state and your gut health.

Creating a mindful lifestyle extends beyond formal practices. Developing a gratitude practice can enhance positivity and shift your focus toward the good in your life. Each day, take a moment to reflect on things you're grateful for, no matter how small. This practice can foster a more optimistic outlook, reducing stress and promoting emotional balance. Engaging in mindful walking or other mindful activities is another way to integrate mindfulness into your life. As you walk, pay attention to the sensations in your body, the rhythm of your breath, and the world around you. This practice can ground you in the present moment, offering a respite from the busyness of daily life.

By embracing mindfulness, you open the door to a world of possibilities for enhancing your gut health and overall well-being. The practices outlined in this chapter are more than just techniques; they are tools for transformation. As you weave mindfulness into your daily routine, you'll find that it not only supports your gut health but also enriches your life in ways you may not have expected. This mindful approach to living is a step toward a more balanced and harmonious existence, setting the stage for the next chapter where we explore overcoming common gut challenges.

6

OVERCOMING COMMON GUT CHALLENGES

P icture this: you're sitting in a crowded room, feeling like a balloon ready to burst. Your stomach is tight, your discomfort is rising, and all you can think about is how to escape this awkward situation. Bloating and gas, those unwelcome companions, can strike at the most inconvenient times, leaving you self-conscious and uncomfortable. You're not alone. Many people experience these symptoms regularly, and they can stem from a variety of sources. Understanding the causes and learning how to tackle them can transform your day-to-day life, allowing you to move through the world with confidence and ease.

6.1 TACKLING BLOATING AND GAS: EFFECTIVE REMEDIES

Bloating and gas are often the result of common dietary and lifestyle choices. One frequent cause is the excessive consumption of high-fiber foods. While fiber is crucial for a healthy diet, consuming too much too quickly can over-whelm your digestive system, leading to bloating. Foods like beans, lentils, and certain vegetables are rich in fiber and can be culprits if not introduced gradually. Another cause is swallowing air, which can happen when you eat too quickly or drink carbonated beverages. These behaviors can trap air in your digestive tract, causing that familiar bloated feeling and excessive gas. It's like a balloon being inflated inside you, creating pressure and discomfort.

To alleviate these symptoms, consider making some dietary adjustments. One effective strategy is to reduce your intake of high-FODMAP foods. These foods, which include onions, garlic, and certain fruits, can ferment in the gut and produce gas. By reducing these foods, you may find relief from bloating. Increasing your water intake can also aid digestion. Water helps move food through the digestive tract, preventing constipation and reducing bloating. It's a simple yet powerful way to keep your system running smoothly. Imagine your digestive system as a well-oiled machine, where water acts as the lubricant that keeps everything functioning without a hitch.

Natural remedies can provide additional support in managing bloating and gas. Peppermint tea, known for its soothing properties, can relax the digestive muscles and reduce bloating. It acts as a gentle balm, easing discomfort and promoting digestion. Activated charcoal supplements are another option. They work by trapping gas-producing compounds in the gut, reducing bloating and gas. These supplements, often available in capsule form, can be a valuable addition to your digestive toolkit. However, it's wise to consult with a healthcare provider before starting any supplement, ensuring it's appropriate for your individual needs.

Embracing mindful eating practices can prevent bloating from occurring in the first place. By slowing down and being present during meals, you can reduce the likelihood of swallowing air. Chewing your food thoroughly aids digestion, breaking down food particles and allowing enzymes to work more effectively. This simple act can make a significant difference in how you feel after eating. Taking smaller bites and savoring each mouthful can also help, reducing air intake and promoting better digestion. It's about creating a mindful dining experience, where each meal becomes an opportunity to nourish your body and support your gut health.

Reflection Section: Mindful Eating Exercise

To practice mindful eating, start by setting aside time for a distraction-free meal. Turn off your phone, step away from your desk, and focus solely on your food. Take a moment to appreciate the colors, textures, and aromas on your plate. As you eat, chew each bite slowly and thoroughly, noticing the flavors and sensations. Pay attention to your body's signals, recognizing when you feel satisfied rather than full. This exercise can help you develop a deeper connection with your food, reducing bloating and enhancing your overall dining experience. Try this practice for a week and reflect on any changes in your digestive comfort and awareness.

6.2 MANAGING FOOD SENSITIVITIES: LISTEN TO YOUR BODY

Navigating the world of food sensitivities can feel like walking a tightrope, where one misstep leads to discomfort or fatigue. Unlike food allergies, which involve an immediate immune response and can be severe, food sensitivities are more subtle. They don't provoke the immune system in the same way but can still cause significant symptoms. Bloating, headaches, and fatigue are common indicators that your body isn't thrilled with something you've eaten. Yet, these reactions aren't as straightforward as allergies, making them trickier to pin down. Intolerances, like lactose intolerance, occur when your body lacks the enzymes to digest certain foods, leading to discomfort but not an immune response. Understanding these distinctions is vital in identifying what might be affecting you.

Identifying your personal triggers requires a bit of detective work. It's about tuning into your body's signals and understanding the language it speaks. One effective method is keeping a food diary. By meticulously recording what you eat and any symptoms that follow, patterns may emerge. This practice requires patience and honesty with yourself, as it involves tracking everything from meals to snacks and even beverages. Over time, you'll be able to see connections between specific foods and how they make you feel, providing valuable insights into your body's preferences. Another approach is an elimination diet, where you remove certain foods from your diet for a period, then gradually reintroduce them. This method helps isolate problematic foods, giving you clarity on what to avoid. With each reintroduction, you can assess how your body responds, gaining a deeper understanding of its needs and sensitivities.

Once you've identified the foods that don't sit well with you, finding alternatives becomes paramount. If lactose is a culprit, fear not; there are plenty of lactose-free options available. Lactose-free milk, cheese, and yogurt are widely accessible, allowing you to enjoy dairy without the discomfort. For those sensitive to gluten, grains like quinoa and rice offer excellent substitutes. These grains are naturally gluten-free, providing versatility in cooking while ensuring you don't miss out on essential nutrients. They can be used in salads, stir-fries, or as side dishes, seamlessly integrating into your meals. Exploring these alternatives not only alleviates symptoms but also expands your culinary repertoire, introducing you to new flavors and textures that support your body's needs.

Personalized nutrition is the cornerstone of managing food sensitivities effectively. Generic dietary advice can only take you so far, as each individual's needs are unique. Consulting with a nutritionist can provide tailored guidance, helping you navigate the complexities of your diet with expert advice. A nutritionist can offer insights into nutrient deficiencies that may arise from eliminating certain foods and suggest ways to maintain a balanced diet. Listening to your body is equally important. It communicates in subtle ways, signaling when something isn't right. By paying attention to these cues and adjusting your diet accordingly, you can foster a harmonious relationship with food. This approach empowers you to make informed choices that align with your body's specific requirements, enhancing your overall well-being.

Interactive Element: Food Sensitivity Tracker

Create a personalized food sensitivity tracker to help identify your triggers. Use a notebook or digital tool to log your meals, noting any symptoms that occur throughout the day. Include details such as the time of day, portion sizes, and any beverages consumed. After a few weeks, review your entries to spot potential patterns. Are there specific foods that consistently correlate with discomfort? Use this information to make informed decisions about your diet, eliminating or substituting foods as needed. This exercise encourages mindfulness and provides a clearer picture of how your body responds to different foods, supporting your path toward better health.

6.3 REGULARITY AND BALANCE: SOLVING DIGESTIVE WOES

Imagine starting your day feeling light and refreshed, without the nagging discomfort of irregular digestion. Unfortunately, many people struggle with this issue, often due to common but overlooked factors. One major culprit is low fiber intake. Fiber is like the unsung hero of digestion, keeping things moving smoothly through your system. Without enough fiber, you might find yourself dealing with constipation, where bowel movements become infrequent or difficult to pass. This can lead to a feeling of heaviness and discomfort. Another factor is dehydration. When your body lacks water, stool can become hard and difficult to pass, exacerbating issues of irregularity. It's like trying to navigate a river without enough water to carry the current; things quickly come to a standstill.

To improve regularity, consider incorporating more soluble fiber into your diet. Soluble fiber, found in foods like oats and apples, acts like a sponge, absorbing water and forming a gel-like substance that eases the passage of stool. This type of fiber not only promotes regular bowel movements but also helps maintain healthy cholesterol levels. Oats can be a comforting breakfast option, while apples make for a convenient snack that supports your digestion. Alongside fiber, make sure you're drinking adequate water. Hydration is key to keeping your digestive system functioning properly. Water helps break down food, absorb nutrients, and soften stool, making it easier to pass. Aim for at least eight glasses a day, and consider more if you're active or live in a hot climate.

Physical activity plays a crucial role in enhancing digestive regularity. When you move, so does your digestive system. Walking after a meal can stimulate digestion, helping food move through your system more efficiently. It's a simple yet effective way to support your gut health, especially if you make it a regular part of your routine. Yoga is another excellent practice for promoting regularity. Certain yoga poses, like twists and forward bends, are known to massage the internal organs and promote bowel movements. Incorporating a few minutes of yoga into your daily routine can have a profound impact on your digestion, providing both physical and mental relaxation.

Establishing consistent routines is vital for maintaining digestive health. Your body thrives on regularity, and setting fixed meal times can help regulate your digestion. When you eat at the same times each day, your body learns to anticipate meals and prepare for digestion, optimizing nutrient absorption and bowel movements. Developing a morning routine that includes time for bathroom use is also beneficial. Just like training any muscle, your digestive system responds well to routine. By setting aside time each morning to relax and allow for a bowel movement, you create a predictable pattern that encourages regularity. This approach not only supports your physical health but also sets a positive tone for the day ahead.

Living a life with regular digestion means feeling more comfortable and confident in your body. You don't have to accept irregularity as the norm. By making small changes to your diet, incorporating movement, and establishing routines, you can support your body's natural processes and enjoy the benefits of a well-functioning digestive system. It's about creating a lifestyle that aligns with your body's needs, fostering a sense of balance and wellbeing that permeates all aspects of your life.

6.4 FATIGUE FIGHTERS: REVITALIZING ENERGY LEVELS

Think of your body as a finely tuned engine. To keep it running smoothly, you need both quality fuel and regular maintenance. When your gut isn't functioning properly, it can feel like trying to drive on an empty tank. Fatigue and low energy levels are common signals that something's amiss in your digestive system. Often, the culprit is nutrient malabsorption. If your gut isn't absorbing nutrients effectively, your body can't produce the energy it needs to keep you going. This can lead to persistent tiredness, no matter how much sleep you get or how many cups of coffee you drink. Gut inflammation can also sap your energy. When your gut is inflamed, it diverts energy away from other bodily functions to focus on healing, leaving you feeling drained and sluggish.

To boost your energy levels, focus on dietary strategies that support gut health. Start by incorporating complex carbohydrates into your meals. Unlike simple carbs, which provide a quick but fleeting energy boost, complex carbohydrates offer sustained energy. Foods like whole grains, sweet potatoes, and brown rice release energy slowly, giving you a steady supply throughout the day. They're like a slow-burning log on a fire, keeping the flames alive without the risk of burning out too quickly. Including iron-rich foods in your diet is also crucial. Iron plays a vital role in oxygen transport, and without enough, you might feel fatigued and weak. Spinach, lentils, and lean meats are excellent sources of iron, helping to replenish your body's stores and boost your energy.

Lifestyle changes can make a significant difference in combating fatigue. Prioritize sleep and rest to allow your body to restore its energy reserves. Aim for a consistent sleep schedule, going to bed and waking up at the same time each day, even on weekends. This routine helps regulate your body's internal clock, ensuring you wake up feeling refreshed. It's also essential to balance work and leisure. Overloading yourself with tasks can lead to burnout, leaving you with little energy for the things you enjoy. Make time for activities that relax and recharge you, whether it's reading a book, going for a walk, or spending time with loved ones. These breaks are not just a luxury; they're a necessity for maintaining vitality.

Hydration plays an often-underestimated role in energy levels. Dehydration can lead to fatigue, as your body struggles to perform basic functions without enough water. Make a habit of drinking water throughout the day, not just when you feel thirsty. Carry a water bottle with you as a reminder to sip regularly. In addition to water, consume hydrating foods like cucumbers and watermelon. These foods are high in water content and can contribute to your overall hydration. Their refreshing nature makes them perfect snacks for a quick energy boost, especially during hot weather.

By addressing these areas, you can create a foundation for sustained energy and vitality. It's about nourishing your body with the right foods, getting enough rest, and making lifestyle choices that support your overall wellbeing. When your gut is healthy, your energy levels naturally follow suit, allowing you to tackle each day with enthusiasm and vigor.

In this chapter, we've explored practical solutions for common gut challenges, from managing bloating to enhancing energy levels. Each strategy is a piece of the puzzle, contributing to a well-functioning digestive system and a healthier you. As you implement these changes, remember that small adjustments can lead to significant improvements. In the next chapter, we'll delve into age-specific gut health solutions, offering tailored advice for different life stages.

7

AGE-SPECIFIC GUT HEALTH SOLUTIONS

I n the whirlwind of adolescence, between school, social activities, and blossoming independence, your gut might not seem like a top priority. However, these formative years lay the groundwork for lifelong health, making it crucial to pay attention to what you eat and how you live. Picture your body as a house under construction. The foundation you lay now will determine its strength and stability for years to come. Establishing healthy habits during your teenage years can fortify this foundation, ensuring a resilient and robust gut that supports you through life's many stages.

7.1 TEENS AND GUT HEALTH: BUILDING FOUNDATIONS

Teens, this is the perfect time to experiment with different fruits and vegetables. Your body is growing and changing, and it needs a diverse range of nutrients to support this development. Think of it as a colorful palette; the more colors you include, the more vibrant your health will be. Embrace the greens of spinach and kale, the reds of tomatoes and strawberries, the yellows of peppers and bananas. Each hue represents a unique set of vitamins and minerals that can enhance your gut health. Avoid relying solely on fast food or sugary snacks. These may be convenient or tempting but can lead to imbalances in your gut microbiome, potentially affecting digestion and mood over time. Source 2 indicates that a diet high in processed foods can reduce gut microbiota diversity, impacting your overall wellbeing.

Nutritional needs during adolescence are unique. Your bones are growing rapidly, requiring ample calcium and vitamin D. Dairy products, leafy greens, and fortified cereals can help meet these needs, supporting both bone and gut health. Balancing meals might seem challenging with a busy schedule, but it doesn't have to be. Consider preparing simple, nutritious snacks that you can grab on the go, like yogurt with fruit or a handful of nuts. These choices ensure you're fueling your body with the nutrients it needs without sacrificing convenience. And remember, breakfast is key. It kickstarts your metabolism and provides energy for the day ahead, so don't skip it! Opt for whole grains and proteins to keep you full and focused.

Social dynamics play a significant role in shaping dietary choices during these years. Peer pressure can lead you to make choices that aren't always the best for your gut. Whether it's indulging in too many sugary drinks at a party or skipping meals because it's the "cool" thing to do, these habits can disrupt your digestive health. When attending gatherings, aim for balance. Enjoy the treats, but also seek out healthier options when available. Communicate your dietary preferences with friends. You might be surprised at how supportive they can be. This openness not only reinforces your commitment to health but also encourages others to consider their own choices.

Mindful eating is a powerful practice to cultivate during adolescence. It's about slowing down, savoring each bite, and really listening to your body. Pay attention to how different foods make you feel. Are you energized or sluggish? Full or still hungry? By tuning into these signals, you can develop a healthier relationship with food, one that supports your gut and overall wellbeing. Techniques like chewing slowly and putting your fork down between bites can enhance digestion and allow your brain to catch up with your stomach, helping you recognize when you're truly satisfied.

Reflection Section: Mindful Eating Journal

Start a mindful eating journal. Note what you eat, when you eat, and how you feel afterward. Record any patterns you notice, such as certain foods that energize you or those that leave you feeling bloated. This practice can provide valuable insights into your eating habits, empowering you to make informed choices that benefit your gut and overall health.

7.2 YOUNG ADULTS: NAVIGATING STRESS AND GUT BALANCE

As you step into young adulthood, life picks up its pace. It's a whirlwind of career ambitions, social commitments, and the newfound responsibilities of independence. These changes can take a toll on your gut health, often leaving you feeling a bit off balance. Amidst the chaos, finding time for meal prep might seem like a luxury, but it's a game-changer for maintaining energy and gut balance. By dedicating just a few hours each week to prepare meals, you ensure that you're not reaching for sugary snacks or fast food when hunger strikes. Consider batching dishes like grain bowls or salads that keep well in the fridge. This way, you have quick, nutritious options at your fingertips, making it easier to eat regularly and support your digestive system.

Stress becomes a constant companion in young adulthood, whether from deadlines at work or navigating new social landscapes. Managing this stress is crucial for both mental and gut health. Incorporate short meditation sessions into your daily routine. Even a few minutes of focused breathing can calm the mind and soothe the gut. Physical activities like yoga or running offer another layer of relief. They help release tension, promote endorphins, and keep your body moving in a way that supports digestion. The rhythm of running or the flow of yoga can help you find moments of peace amidst a hectic schedule.

Sleep often becomes a casualty of a busy lifestyle, yet it's vital for maintaining gut health and overall wellbeing. Sleep is when your body repairs and restores itself, including your digestive system. Without enough rest, your gut can become more permeable, leading to imbalances. Creating a consistent sleep schedule can help. Aim for seven to nine hours a night, going to bed and waking up at the same time. Improving sleep hygiene is also key. Turn off screens an hour before bed, keep your room cool and dark, and consider a wind-down routine that relaxes your mind and body.

Young adulthood is also a time when dietary pitfalls are easy to stumble into. Caffeine and alcohol often become staples, but they can disrupt gut health if not managed carefully. Caffeine can lead to stomach irritation and anxiety, so try limiting your intake to one or two cups of coffee a day. Alcohol, while a social lubricant, can harm the gut lining and should be consumed in moderation. Instead, choose whole foods over fast food. Whole foods, such as fruits, vegetables, and lean proteins, provide the nutrients that processed foods lack. They nourish your body and support a healthy microbiome, helping you feel your best even when life gets hectic.

Navigating young adulthood is about finding balance amidst change. By making mindful choices—whether through meal prepping, stress management, sleep, or diet—you can support your gut and thrive in this dynamic phase of life.

7.3 MIDLIFE ADJUSTMENTS: ADAPTING TO CHANGES

As you reach midlife, you might notice that your body doesn't quite respond to things the way it used to. This is a time when subtle yet significant physiological changes can affect your gut health. One of the most noticeable shifts is a slowing metabolism, which can make digestion less efficient. This change often leads to increased instances of constipation, a common yet uncomfortable issue. To combat this, increasing your fiber intake becomes crucial. Foods like whole grains, legumes, fruits, and vegetables are rich in fiber and can help keep things moving smoothly through your digestive tract. Incorporating these foods into your meals not only aids digestion but also supports a healthy microbiome, which is vital for overall gut health.

Hormonal changes during midlife, such as those experienced during menopause or andropause, can also have a profound impact on your gut. These shifts can lead to symptoms like bloating, indigestion, and changes in bowel habits. For those experiencing menopause, dietary adjustments can help manage these symptoms. Including foods rich in phytoestrogens, such as soy products, flaxseeds, and chickpeas, can support hormonal balance and potentially ease digestive discomfort. Phytoestrogens are plant compounds that mimic the effects of estrogen in the body, helping to stabilize hormone levels naturally. By making these dietary choices, you can navigate the hormonal rollercoaster with a bit more ease and promote a healthier gut environment.

Maintaining a healthy weight in midlife can feel like an uphill battle, particularly with a metabolism that seems to have hit the brakes. However, it's entirely possible with a few strategic adjustments. Portion control becomes more important than ever. By being mindful of serving sizes and focusing on balanced meals, you can manage your weight more effectively. This approach helps prevent overeating and ensures that your body gets the nutrients it needs without excess calories. Regular physical activity is another cornerstone of weight management. It doesn't have to be strenuous—activities like brisk walking, swimming, or cycling can work wonders. Exercise not only boosts metabolism but also enhances digestion and improves mood, making it a win-win for your gut and overall health.

Routine health check-ups become even more valuable as you progress through midlife. These visits are an opportunity to monitor your gut health and address any concerns before they become more serious. Screening for common gastrointestinal issues, such as diverticulosis or acid reflux, can provide peace of mind and guide you in making necessary lifestyle adjustments. During these check-ups, don't hesitate to discuss any gut health concerns with your healthcare provider. Whether it's changes in bowel habits or persistent digestive discomfort, these discussions can lead to valuable insights and tailored advice. Proactively managing your health in this way can help you maintain a vibrant and active life, even as your body undergoes natural changes.

By understanding these midlife adjustments and implementing thoughtful strategies, you can continue to enjoy a life full of vitality and wellness. Your gut health plays a significant role in this, acting as a foundation for overall wellbeing.

7.4 SENIORS: MAINTAINING GUT VITALITY

As you grow older, your body's needs begin to shift, and nowhere is this more evident than in the gut. Nutrient absorption changes with age, making a nutrient-rich diet more important than ever. Vitamins B12 and D are crucial. B12 supports nerve function and the production of DNA, while vitamin D enhances calcium absorption, crucial for bone health. However, as the stomach lining thins with age, B12 absorption can decrease, leading to deficiencies. To combat this, include fortified foods like cereals and plant milks, or discuss supplements with your healthcare provider.

Protein is another key player. It helps maintain muscle mass, which tends to decline as you age. Incorporate lean sources of protein such as fish, legumes, and eggs into your meals to keep your muscles strong and your gut content.

Digestive issues are common among seniors, with constipation and dehydration among the most prevalent. Constipation can be uncomfortable and lead to other health complications if not managed properly. To alleviate this, ensure you're consuming enough fiber-rich foods, including fruits, vegetables, and whole grains. These foods help maintain regular bowel movements. Hydration is equally important. As you age, the sensation of thirst diminishes, increasing the risk of dehydration, which can exacerbate constipation. Aiming for at least eight glasses of water a day can keep your digestive system running smoothly. Herbal teas and broths can also be soothing and hydrating alternatives, making it easier to meet your fluid needs.

Staying active is essential for maintaining gut health and vitality as you age. Physical activity helps maintain digestive regularity and overall well-being. Gentle exercises like tai chi or walking can be particularly beneficial. Tai chi, with its slow and deliberate movements, not only improves balance and flexibility but also promotes relaxation, which can positively impact gut health. Walking is a simple yet effective way to keep your body moving, and it can be easily adapted to suit different fitness levels. Participating in social activities that encourage movement, such as group fitness classes or dance sessions, can also provide a sense of community and motivation, making exercise enjoyable and sustainable.

Social interactions and communal meals play a significant role in promoting digestive health and overall well-being for seniors. Participating in community meal programs can offer both nutritional benefits and social engagement, reducing feelings of isolation and providing opportunities to enjoy balanced, nutritious meals with others. These programs can introduce you to new foods and recipes, expanding your culinary repertoire and supporting gut health. Hosting regular family dinners or gatherings with friends can also foster connection and encourage healthy eating habits. Sharing meals with loved ones not only strengthens relationships but also creates an environment where you can enjoy a variety of foods that support your digestive system.

Maintaining gut vitality in your later years involves understanding and addressing the unique nutritional needs and challenges that come with aging. By focusing on a nutrient-rich diet, managing common digestive issues, staying active, and fostering social connections through communal meals, you can support a healthy gut and enjoy a vibrant, fulfilling life. These strategies not only promote digestive health but also contribute to overall well-being, allowing you to embrace the joys of aging with confidence and vitality. As we wrap up this chapter, consider how these age-specific solutions fit into the larger picture of holistic health.

8

ADDRESSING SOCIAL AND RELATIONSHIP DYNAMICS

When I first started making changes to improve my gut health, I didn't anticipate how it would affect my social life. Picture yourself at a family dinner, where the table is laden with all your favorite dishes. You find yourself hesitating, unsure how to explain to your aunt why you're skipping the creamy pasta or the rich chocolate cake. It's not just about the food—it's about sharing a part of your life that feels deeply personal. Yet, it's this very openness that can transform your health journey from an isolated endeavor into a shared experience.

8.1 Communicating Your Health Journey

Open communication is a bridge that connects your internal changes with the world around you. Sharing your health journey with friends and family can be daunting, but it is crucial for creating a supportive environment. When you articulate your experiences and goals, you invite others to understand and perhaps join you in making healthier choices. However, the idea of laying bare such personal details can be intimidating, especially if you're worried about judgment or misunderstanding. It's natural to feel hesitant about opening up, but overcoming this initial reluctance is the first step toward fostering empathy and support.

Choosing the right time and setting for these conversations can make all the difference. A quiet moment during a one-on-one chat may offer a more receptive atmosphere than a bustling family gathering. When you feel ready to share, frame your conversation around your personal experiences using "I" statements. This approach helps convey that these changes are about your health and wellbeing, not a critique of others' choices. Instead of focusing on restrictions, emphasize the benefits you're experiencing, like increased energy or reduced discomfort. This positive framing can encourage curiosity rather than defensiveness.

Effective communication is a two-way street, and empathy plays a vital role. Encourage your loved ones to ask questions and express their thoughts. Engaging in open-ended questions can facilitate meaningful dialogue and demonstrate your willingness to listen. For instance, ask them what they know about gut health or if they've noticed any changes in their own wellbeing. These questions can open up a conversation that feels inclusive and collaborative. Demonstrating patience and understanding during discussions, even when faced with skepticism, can prevent conversations from becoming confrontational. Remember, everyone processes information differently, and some may need time to fully grasp the significance of your choices.

Handling difficult conversations requires a calm and composed approach. You might encounter resistance or skepticism, especially if your changes challenge long-held family traditions or beliefs. Responding with facts and personal experiences rather than defensiveness can help alleviate doubts. Share statistics or personal anecdotes that highlight the benefits of your lifestyle adjustments. Your journey is unique, and sharing your story can sometimes be more persuasive than any research article. If negative comments arise, maintain your composure and remember that your health is the priority. It's okay to set boundaries, reminding others that while you're open to discussing your choices, you're also committed to what works best for you.

Reflection Section: Open Dialogue Checklist

Consider using a checklist to prepare for these conversations:

1. Identify key points you want to convey about your health journey.
2. Choose a time and setting that feels comfortable and conducive to open dialogue.

3. Practice using "I" statements to express your experiences and goals.
4. Prepare to engage with empathy, asking open-ended questions to encourage discussion.
5. Plan responses to potential skepticism, including personal anecdotes or facts.

Through open and empathetic communication, you can cultivate a supportive network that understands and encourages your health journey. This dialogue not only strengthens your relationships but also reinforces your commitment to a healthier, more balanced lifestyle.

8.2 OVERCOMING JUDGMENT AND STIGMA

Navigating the world of gut health can sometimes feel like venturing into uncharted territory, especially when societal perceptions come into play. It's not unusual to encounter raised eyebrows or curious glances when you make significant lifestyle changes, particularly those involving dietary restrictions or unconventional health choices. The stigma associated with altering your diet can stem from a lack of understanding or deeply ingrained cultural norms. For some, the idea of excluding certain foods is seen as a fad or an unnecessary inconvenience, rather than a genuine effort to improve health. This misunderstanding can lead to social awkwardness or even judgment, making it challenging to stay confident in your choices. But it's important to remember that these changes are deeply personal and rooted in your well-being.

Building resilience against judgment requires a strong sense of self and confidence in your decisions. A personal mantra or affirmation can serve as a reminder of your goals and the reasons behind your choices. Something as simple as repeating, "I am prioritizing my health," can anchor you in moments of doubt or criticism. Engaging in self-reflection is another powerful tool. Take time to revisit your personal goals and remind yourself why you embarked on this path. Reflecting on your progress and the benefits you've experienced can reinforce your commitment and help you maintain focus despite any external noise. This inner strength is crucial for navigating social settings where dietary changes might draw attention.

Education plays a key role in reducing the stigma surrounding gut health choices. Often, misunderstandings arise from a lack of knowledge about why someone might choose to alter their diet or lifestyle. By sharing informative articles or resources with those who are genuinely curious, you can help dismantle stereotypes and foster acceptance. Consider hosting small gatherings where you can openly discuss your health journey and the reasons behind your decisions. These intimate settings provide an opportunity to educate others and dispel myths in a relaxed and personal environment. It's about creating a dialogue that encourages curiosity and learning, rather than judgment.

Maintaining relationships despite differing health perspectives can be challenging but not impossible. Agreeing to disagree on certain topics can preserve harmony, allowing you and your loved ones to coexist with respect for each other's choices. It's important to find common ground in shared interests beyond health. Whether it's a mutual love for a hobby, a favorite movie, or family traditions, these connections can strengthen bonds and remind everyone that while health choices might differ, the relationship remains intact. By focusing on what unites you rather than what separates you, you can maintain meaningful connections without compromising your health priorities.

Reflection Section: Navigating Judgment and Stigma

Consider these prompts to reflect on your experiences with judgment:

1. What misconceptions about your health choices have you encountered?
2. How have you responded to judgment or misunderstanding in the past?
3. Identify a personal mantra or affirmation that reinforces your commitment to your health.
4. List ways you can educate others about your choices, such as sharing resources or hosting discussions.
5. Reflect on common interests you share with loved ones that can strengthen your relationships despite differing health views.

8.3 FINDING SUPPORT IN SOCIAL CIRCLES

Navigating the path to better health is often smoother with a supportive network by your side. Having family and friends who understand and encourage you can make all the difference. Emotional support can act as a cushion during challenging times, offering reassurance and motivation when you need it most. Picture your friends as a team, cheering you on from the sidelines. Their presence can fuel your journey, reminding you that you're not alone in your pursuit of better health. A network of supportive peers can also foster accountability. Knowing there are people who care about your progress can motivate you to stay on track with your goals. Even a simple check-in from a friend can serve as a gentle nudge, encouraging you to continue making healthy choices.

Recognizing supportive individuals in your life involves looking for certain traits and behaviors. Supportive people are open-minded and willing to learn about your experiences. They're the ones who ask questions and show genuine interest in your health goals. They offer consistent encouragement, celebrating your successes and providing a listening ear when challenges arise. Positive reinforcement from these individuals can boost your confidence, reinforcing the belief that you're making meaningful strides toward better health. These allies are invaluable, providing a sense of stability and reassurance as you navigate the ups and downs of your health journey.

Cultivating support within existing relationships involves nurturing these bonds. Sharing your successes and progress regularly can strengthen these connections. When you share your achievements, you're inviting your loved ones to be part of your journey, fostering a sense of camaraderie and shared purpose. Consider inviting friends and family to participate in health-related activities with you. Whether it's a weekend hike, a cooking class, or a yoga session, these shared experiences can deepen your connections and create lasting memories. By involving your loved ones in your health pursuits, you reinforce the importance of collaboration and mutual support.

Expanding your support network beyond immediate social circles can introduce you to new perspectives and friendships. Joining online communities focused on gut health can connect you with like-minded individuals who share your interests and challenges. These virtual spaces offer a platform for exchanging ideas, sharing tips, and finding solace in shared experiences. Participating in local wellness groups or workshops is another avenue for expanding your network. These gatherings provide an opportunity to meet people who are also committed to living healthier lives. Engaging with others who prioritize wellness can inspire you and offer fresh insights into your own health journey.

Building a strong support system is like gathering a team of allies, each contributing their unique strengths and perspectives. Whether it's your family cheering you on, friends joining you in health activities, or new acquaintances sharing their own stories, each connection adds value to your life. Embrace these relationships and nurture them, knowing they offer both encouragement and accountability as you continue to prioritize your health. A supportive network not only enriches your journey but also reminds you that health is a shared endeavor, strengthened by the bonds we form along the way.

8.4 BUILDING A COMMUNITY OF WELLNESS

Imagine stepping into a room where everyone shares a common goal of better health and wellbeing. This is the essence of a wellness community—a place where camaraderie grows from shared experiences and mutual aspirations. Being part of such a group offers more than just support; it provides a sense of belonging that can motivate and inspire. Within these communities, you find people who understand your challenges and celebrate your successes. The collective knowledge and diversity of experiences present opportunities for learning and growth, allowing you to see your health journey from different perspectives.

Creating or joining a wellness community starts with identifying a common interest or focus. Whether it's gut health, fitness, or mindfulness, the key is to find a topic that resonates with you and potential members. Once this focus is established, consider setting up regular meetings or virtual check-ins. These gatherings can be as simple as a monthly coffee catch-up or an online video chat. Consistent interaction helps maintain momentum, keeping everyone engaged and committed to their health goals.

Engagement is the lifeblood of any community. To keep things dynamic, consider hosting monthly challenges or themed activities. These could range from a week of trying new healthy recipes to a mindfulness challenge where members practice meditation daily. Encouraging members to share personal stories and tips can also foster a sense of connection and understanding. When people openly discuss their experiences, they inspire others and reinforce the community's supportive atmosphere.

In today's digital age, technology plays a crucial role in building and sustaining wellness communities. Creating a private social media group can facilitate discussions, share resources, and provide a space for members to connect outside of regular meetings. These online platforms offer convenience and accessibility, allowing members to participate no matter where they are. Video conferencing tools can further enhance this interaction by enabling virtual meetups. These digital gatherings can mimic the feel of an in-person meeting, making it easier to maintain personal connections and group dynamics.

As you think about building your wellness community, consider the diverse tools at your disposal. From social media groups to video calls, technology allows you to bring people together, fostering a vibrant and supportive environment. This community not only enriches your personal health journey but also contributes to the collective well-being of its members, creating a ripple effect that extends beyond the group itself.

In this chapter, we've delved into the power of wellness communities and their role in fostering health and connection. By creating spaces that nurture shared goals and experiences, we lay the groundwork for collective growth and understanding. As we move forward, let's explore how these principles can extend into broader aspects of life, enhancing not just our health but our overall sense of purpose and belonging.

9

SCIENTIFIC INSIGHTS AND HOLISTIC PRACTICES

P icture yourself as a detective, piecing together clues about your health. Each meal, each emotion, each lifestyle choice contributes to the story of your wellbeing. And at the heart of this mystery lies your gut. It's not just a digestive powerhouse; it's a complex system influencing your mood, immunity, and overall vitality. This chapter dives into the latest scientific research, revealing how your gut can be both a source of problems and solutions. With groundbreaking studies and fascinating discoveries, you're about to see just how pivotal the gut is in maintaining health.

9.1 EVIDENCE-BASED GUT HEALTH: WHAT SCIENCE SAYS

Recent research has unveiled the gut as a central player in preventing diseases. Scientists have found that the gut microbiota—a bustling community of trillions of microorganisms—acts as a gatekeeper, keeping harmful pathogens at bay and modulating the immune system. One key study highlighted the role of specific bacteria in reducing inflammation, a common thread in many chronic diseases. These bacteria produce short-chain fatty acids (SCFAs) that help regulate the immune response, preventing it from going into overdrive and causing harm. This discovery underscores the importance of a balanced microbiota, not just for digestion but as a cornerstone of disease prevention.

The gut-brain axis has received a lot of attention lately, and for good reason. This complex communication network between the gut and the brain influences everything from mood to cognitive function. Recent studies have shown that alterations in gut microbiota can affect neurotransmitter levels, impacting mood disorders like depression and anxiety. The vagus nerve, a major component of this axis, acts as a highway for signals between the gut and brain. It's fascinating to see how what starts in your gut can affect your thoughts and feelings, highlighting the need for gut health in emotional wellbeing.

To ensure the reliability and validity of these findings, researchers employ rigorous methodologies. One common approach is the double-blind placebo-controlled trial, where neither the participants nor the researchers know who receives the treatment or placebo. This method minimizes bias and strengthens the credibility of the results. Longitudinal studies are also crucial, tracking gut health over extended periods to observe changes and long-term effects. These studies help us understand how gut health evolves and its impact on overall wellbeing, offering insights that can guide personal health decisions.

Genetics also play a significant role in shaping your gut health. Twin studies have revealed that genetic predispositions can influence microbiome composition and function. Identical twins, who share the same genetic makeup, often have more similar gut microbiota than fraternal twins, suggesting a genetic component to gut health. This knowledge has paved the way for personalized nutrition, where genetic testing can provide tailored dietary recommendations. By understanding your genetic profile, you can make more informed choices about your diet, optimizing your gut health based on your unique needs.

Translating these scientific insights into actionable advice is where the magic happens. Incorporating fiber-rich foods into your diet is a powerful way to enhance gut bacteria diversity. Foods like lentils, beans, and whole grains are rich in fiber, serving as fuel for beneficial bacteria. Evidence-based probiotics, tailored to specific health conditions, can also support a balanced microbiome. Whether you're dealing with digestive issues or looking to boost your mood, choosing the right probiotics can make a world of difference.

Interactive Element: Personalized Gut Health Plan

Reflect on your current diet and lifestyle. Consider incorporating more fiber-rich foods into your meals. Keep a journal for a week, noting any changes in digestion or mood. Explore genetic testing options to tailor your diet further. This personalized approach empowers you to take charge of your gut health, transforming scientific insights into practical strategies.

9.2 INTEGRATING EASTERN AND WESTERN PHILOSOPHIES

In the realm of gut health, Eastern medicine offers a rich tapestry of insights that have stood the test of time. Take Ayurveda, for instance, which emphasizes balance and harmony. Ayurveda sees the gut as the core of health, tying its function to the balance of the body's energies, known as doshas—Vata, Pitta, and Kapha. These doshas need to be in harmony for optimal health, and any imbalance can lead to digestive issues. This ancient practice prescribes personalized diets, herbal remedies, and lifestyle changes to restore this balance, promoting a healthy digestive "fire" or Agni, which is believed to be crucial for metabolism and vitality.

Traditional Chinese Medicine (TCM) also offers profound insights into gut health. It views the body as an interconnected system where the flow of Qi, or life force, is paramount. In TCM, the spleen and stomach are seen as the center of digestion and energy production. Qi flow must be unobstructed to maintain health, and TCM uses a combination of acupuncture, herbal treatments, and dietary adjustments to ensure this flow remains smooth. These practices aim to strengthen the digestive system, improve nutrient absorption, and prevent the buildup of toxins, which are seen as blockages to health.

Western medicine, on the other hand, approaches gut health with a focus on diagnosis and treatment. Through advanced diagnostic tools like endoscopy and colonoscopy, doctors can visualize and assess the condition of the gastrointestinal tract in detail. These tools allow for precise diagnosis of disorders such as ulcers, polyps, and inflammation. Pharmacological interventions, including antacids, antibiotics, and anti-inflammatory medications, are commonly used to manage gut-related disorders. These treatments often provide quick relief from symptoms, targeting the underlying causes with a scientific precision that Eastern practices might not emphasize.

Despite their differences, Eastern and Western philosophies can beautifully complement each other in managing gut health. The integration of herbal remedies from Ayurveda with modern medications can offer a holistic approach, where the soothing properties of herbs enhance the efficacy of pharmaceuticals. For example, ginger, a staple of Ayurvedic medicine, can be used alongside conventional treatments for nausea, offering a natural complement to medications. Similarly, acupuncture, a cornerstone of TCM, can be integrated with lifestyle modifications to enhance digestive health. By stimulating specific points on the body, acupuncture can promote Qi flow, reduce stress, and improve gut function.

Consider the case of an individual struggling with IBS (Irritable Bowel Syndrome). A treatment plan that combines acupuncture with dietary changes can be particularly effective. Acupuncture sessions can alleviate symptoms like bloating and discomfort, while dietary modifications tailored to the individual's needs can address food sensitivities and improve digestion. Another example is using mindfulness meditation alongside medical therapy for gut disorders. Mindfulness practices can reduce stress-induced gut issues, complementing medications that manage symptoms, creating a comprehensive treatment approach that addresses both the mind and body.

This integration of Eastern and Western philosophies offers a balanced path to gut health, drawing on the strengths of both traditions. By embracing the wisdom of ancient practices and the precision of modern medicine, you can cultivate a more harmonious relationship with your gut, fostering resilience and wellbeing that transcend cultural boundaries.

9.3 HOLISTIC HEALING: BEYOND DIET

The path to a healthier gut isn't just paved with good nutrition. It's a tapestry woven with threads of mental, emotional, and physical wellbeing. When you consider gut health holistically, you're not just looking at what you eat but also how you feel and move. Emotional wellbeing plays a crucial role here. Stress and emotional turmoil can disrupt the gut's delicate balance, leading to digestive issues. Ever notice how anxiety can twist your stomach into knots? That's your gut responding to emotional signals. When you nurture your emotional health, whether through meditation or spending time with loved ones, you create a supportive environment for your gut. It's like giving your digestive system a warm, comforting hug, which can help ease symptoms and promote healing.

Physical activity is another powerful ally for gut balance. It's not just about burning calories or building muscle; it's about creating movement that supports digestion. Regular exercise increases blood flow to the digestive organs, enhancing their efficiency. Activities like walking, jogging, or dancing can stimulate your gut, keeping things moving smoothly and preventing sluggishness. But it's not just the physical bene-fits; exercise releases endorphins, those feel-good chemicals that boost mood and reduce stress. This dual impact of physical activity helps maintain a balanced gut, supporting both your physical and mental health. It's a reminder that your body thrives on movement, and your gut is no exception.

Beyond diet and exercise, alternative therapies offer intriguing possibilities for supporting gut health. Aromatherapy is one such practice that can help manage stress-related gut issues. The soothing scents of lavender, chamomile, or peppermint oils can calm the mind and ease digestive discomfort. You might find that inhaling these aromas or using them in a diffuser creates a sense of relaxation that permeates your entire being. Hydrotherapy, another ancient remedy, involves the use of water to stimulate circulation and digestion. A warm bath can relax the muscles and improve blood flow, while a cold shower might invigorate the digestive process. These therapies, though simple, offer gentle ways to support your gut without relying solely on dietary changes.

Mind-body techniques like yoga and tai chi provide a harmonious blend of physical and mental integration that can enhance gut health. Yoga sequences designed for digestion, such as twists and forward bends, help massage the internal organs, promoting better digestion. These poses can relieve bloating and discomfort, giving your gut the gentle encouragement it needs to function optimally. Tai chi, with its flowing movements and meditative focus, offers stress reduction and balance. The rhythmic, deliberate motions help calm the mind and body, fostering a sense of peace that extends to the gut. These practices remind us that the mind and body are interconnected, and nurturing one supports the other.

Incorporating holistic practices into your daily routine doesn't have to be complicated. Consider starting your day with a morning ritual that includes stretching and mindfulness. A few minutes of gentle stretching can awaken your body, while a brief meditation session sets a positive tone for the day. As you move through your day, consider using essential oils as part of a relaxation routine. A drop of lavender oil on your temples or wrists can provide a moment of calm, helping you to maintain a sense of balance amid life's demands. These small, intentional practices create a foundation of holistic health that supports not just your gut, but your entire being.

9.4 MIND-BODY HARMONY: A UNIFIED APPROACH

Imagine your mind and body in perfect sync, each supporting the other in a dance of health and vitality. This is mind-body harmony, a state where mental and physical health are balanced, each enhancing the other. In the context of gut health, achieving this harmony means recognizing the profound interconnectedness of your thoughts, emotions, and physical wellbeing. When you're stressed, your gut feels it. When you're relaxed, your gut relaxes too. This relationship is more than just a coincidence; it's a reflection of how deeply intertwined our mental and physical states truly are.

Mindfulness, a practice of being present and fully engaged in the moment, plays a crucial role in promoting gut health. Through mindful breathing exercises, you can directly influence your gut function. Picture this: as you take a deep breath in, your diaphragm expands, gently massaging your internal organs. This motion helps stimulate the vagus nerve, which connects the gut and brain, promoting relaxation and better digestion. By focusing on your breath, you also give your mind a break from the stresses of daily life, reducing the stress-induced gut issues that many people face. Mindfulness meditation takes this a step further by encouraging a state of mental calm that can lower stress levels, reducing the release of stress hormones like cortisol, which are known to negatively impact gut health.

Achieving mind-body harmony offers tangible health benefits. One of the most significant is the reduction in cortisol levels, the hormone often dubbed the "stress hormone." High cortisol levels can lead to a range of health issues, including weight gain, high blood pressure, and digestive problems. By engaging in mind-body practices, you can help bring these levels down, promoting a sense of calm and balance. This, in turn, enhances the function of the gut barrier, which acts as a protective shield against harmful pathogens and toxins. A strong gut barrier is essential for maintaining overall health, and reducing stress is a key factor in keeping it intact.

To weave mind-body harmony into your daily life, consider setting daily intentions. This practice involves dedicating a few moments each day to focus on what you want to achieve in terms of mind-body connection. It could be as simple as intending to take a mindful walk, where you pay attention to the sights and sounds around you, or dedicating time to meditate and reflect. Participating in activities that integrate both mind and body, such as dance or martial arts, can also be incredibly beneficial. These activities require you to be present, engaging both your physical and mental faculties in a way that promotes harmony. Dancing allows you to express emotions through movement, while martial arts teach discipline and focus, both of which can enhance your overall sense of wellbeing.

As you explore the concept of mind-body harmony, remember that it's a journey unique to each individual. There's no one-size-fits-all approach, and what works for one person may not work for another. The key is to remain open to experimentation, trying different practices to see what resonates with you. By nurturing this balance, you're not just supporting your gut health; you're cultivating a life-style that honors the connection between mind and body, leading to a richer, more vibrant life.

This chapter has touched on the transformative power of mind-body harmony and its impact on gut health. As you move forward, keep these insights close, and let them guide you in creating a balanced, healthy life.

10

ENGAGING WITH YOUR GUT
HEALTH JOURNEY

Think of your gut health journey as a personal project, one that evolves and grows with you. Imagine you're an architect, designing a blueprint for a healthier you, where each step you take contributes to the masterpiece that is your wellbeing. Tracking your progress is the cornerstone of this endeavor, providing a clear map of where you've been, where you are, and where you aim to go. It's not just about the destination; it's about appreciating every small victory along the way.

Monitoring your gut health journey is pivotal for understanding what strategies work best for you. It allows you to identify patterns and triggers, helping you make informed decisions. Have you ever noticed how keeping a record of your habits can unveil unexpected insights? By consistently tracking your diet and symptoms, you might discover that certain foods trigger discomfort or that stress impacts your digestion. This awareness empowers you to adjust your habits, making your path to better health more efficient and personalized.

Various tools are at your disposal to help track your progress. A food diary is a simple yet effective method. By jotting down what you eat and how you feel afterwards, you can spot trends and make necessary changes. In a digital age, mobile apps like Cara Care or mySymptoms Food Diary offer a convenient way to track dietary habits and symptoms, providing visual representations to identify patterns (SOURCE 1). These apps can be especially helpful if you're managing conditions like IBS or following a specific diet. Wearable devices, such as fitness trackers, can also play a role in monitoring physical activity, ensuring you stay active and support your gut health. These tools can be your allies, offering insights and motivation as you move forward.

Setting realistic goals is key to maintaining motivation and ensuring progress. The SMART goal framework—Specific, Measurable, Achievable, Relevant, and Time-bound—provides a structured approach that turns vague aspirations into tangible targets. For instance, instead of saying, "I want to eat healthier," a SMART goal would be, "I will eat at least three servings of vegetables daily for the next month" (SOURCE 4). This precise goal is not only clear and measurable but also achievable and relevant to your broader health objectives. Short-term goals, such as trying a new gut-friendly recipe each week, can keep you engaged and excited. Long-term goals, like cultivating a more balanced micro-biome over six months, ensure you have a vision to strive towards.

Regular assessment of your progress is crucial to stay on track and adapt as needed. Consider scheduling monthly check-ins with yourself. During these check-ins, review your food diary or app logs to evaluate dietary changes. Reflect on your emotional wellbeing and how your gut health might be influencing it. This practice encourages you to adjust your strategies, ensuring they remain effective and aligned with your goals. Reflective journaling can be a valuable tool during these assessments, allowing you to explore your thoughts and feelings, fostering a deeper connection between your mind and gut. By consistently evaluating your progress and making adjustments, you maintain momentum and continue moving towards a healthier, more balanced life.

10.1 PERSONAL STORIES OF TRANSFORMATION

Imagine sitting across from Sarah, a young woman who once battled the relentless discomfort of IBS. Her days were filled with uncertainty, never knowing when her symptoms might flare up. It wasn't until she decided to take control, focusing on dietary changes, that she found relief. Sarah began by eliminating common triggers like gluten and dairy, and introduced a variety of fibrous vegetables and fermented foods into her diet. The transformation wasn't overnight, but with determination and patience, Sarah noticed a significant reduction in her symptoms. Her energy levels soared, and she finally felt in tune with her body. Her story is a testament to the power of dietary choices in reclaiming one's health.

Then there's Alex, whose emotional rollercoaster seemed to have no end. He struggled with anxiety and mood swings that disrupted his relationships and daily life. It wasn't until he began nurturing his gut that things started to change. By incorporating more plant-based meals and practicing mindfulness, Alex found a new level of emotional balance. The mindfulness practices helped him manage stress, while the plant-based diet supported a healthier gut environment. Slowly, Alex discovered a newfound peace and stability, enabling him to engage with life more fully. His journey highlights how interconnected our gut and emotions truly are, and how taking steps to care for one can positively affect the other.

In exploring these stories, we see diverse approaches to gut health. They demonstrate how different strategies can lead to successful outcomes. The impact of a plant-based diet, as seen in Alex's story, shows us how powerful food can be in promoting a balanced microbiome. Meanwhile, incorporating mindfulness practices serves as a gentle reminder of the importance of mental health in the overall equation. These methods are not one-size-fits-all, but rather adaptable to individual needs and preferences, illustrating the flexibility required in personal health journeys.

Challenges are inevitable, and these individuals faced their fair share. Sarah encountered skepticism from her family, who questioned her dietary changes. Yet, she persisted, educating them about her needs and showing them the positive results. Alex had setbacks, moments when stress overwhelmed him, threatening to derail his progress. But he remained committed, using these challenges as opportunities to strengthen his resolve. They both teach us that perseverance is key, and that obstacles, though daunting, are surmountable with the right mindset and support.

Drawing inspiration from these stories can be a powerful motivator. They remind us that we're not alone in our struggles. By identifying common challenges and solutions, you can find a sense of camaraderie and hope. These narratives provide a source of determination, encouraging you to continue pursuing your health goals with confidence. They show that while the path to improved gut health may be challenging, it is also rewarding. Each step forward brings you closer to a healthier, more harmonious life.

Interactive Elements: Engaging with Your Journey

Imagine your gut health journey as an immersive, interactive experience filled with opportunities to actively engage and learn. Interactive elements are like the interactive exhibits at a museum, inviting you to touch, explore, and truly understand the complexity of your body's systems. They can transform the process of improving your gut health from a passive pursuit into a dynamic adventure. Quizzes, for instance, can be a fun way to test your knowledge about gut health. They reinforce what you've learned and highlight areas where you might need a bit more focus. Challenges are another exciting element, pushing you to implement new habits, whether it's trying a new recipe each week or practicing mindfulness regularly. These activities keep you engaged, motivated, and constantly moving forward.

There are numerous engaging activities you can incorporate into your routine to keep things lively and interesting. Weekly meal planning challenges can be a great start. By dedicating some time each week to plan your meals, you ensure they're balanced, nutritious, and tailored to your gut health goals. It's a practical way to apply what you've learned and see real results. Mindfulness meditation sessions, enhanced with guided audio, can help you connect with your body and mind more deeply. These sessions offer a moment of peace in a busy day, reducing stress and supporting your gut. Additionally, participating in group discussions or joining online forums can provide a sense of community. Sharing experiences, tips, and encouragement with others on a similar path can be incredibly empowering. It reminds you that you're not alone and that there's a wealth of wisdom to be gained from others.

The role of community in interactive engagement cannot be overstated. Connecting with others who share your goals can significantly enhance your experience. Online support groups and local wellness workshops or seminars offer platforms for interaction and mutual support. These spaces allow you to share your successes, discuss your challenges, and gain insights from others who are on similar journeys. They foster a sense of accountability, motivating you to stay committed to your health goals. Moreover, the camaraderie found in these groups can provide emotional support, making the process feel less daunting and more like a shared adventure.

Encouraging creativity and personalization in these activities adds another layer of engagement. Personalization means tailoring your approach to fit your unique preferences and needs. For instance, creating personalized vision boards for your health goals can be a powerful visual reminder of what you're working towards. Designing unique tracking systems that resonate with your style can also enhance engagement. These systems might include a combination of digital tools, like apps, alongside more traditional methods, like journaling or checklists. By making the process your own, you ensure it remains relevant and motivating. This personal touch not only keeps you engaged but also makes the journey more enjoyable and meaningful.

10.2 SELF-REFLECTION AND GROWTH

In the hustle and bustle of daily life, it's easy to overlook the power of self-reflection. Yet, taking a moment to look inward can offer profound insights into your health and wellbeing. Self-reflection acts like a mirror, showing you not only where you are but also how far you've come. It allows you to dig deep into your experiences, helping you understand the choices that have brought you to this point. Reflective journaling can be an invaluable tool in this process. By putting pen to paper, you create a tangible record of your thoughts and feelings, offering a safe space for self-discovery. Whether it's noting the foods that make you feel your best or the emotions that arise during stressful times, these reflections serve as a guide to inform future decisions. You can learn from past challenges and use them as stepping stones to progress.

To facilitate introspection, consider asking yourself a few guiding questions. What changes have you noticed in your physical and emotional health? This question encourages you to examine the tangible and intangible shifts that have occurred since you started focusing on your gut health. Another question to ponder is how your perspectives on health have evolved. Reflecting on this can reveal the growth in your understanding and approach to wellness. These questions are not meant to be answered in one sitting; rather, they should be revisited periodically as your journey unfolds. By regularly engaging with these prompts, you create a dialogue with yourself, fostering a deeper connection to your health.

Adopting a growth mindset can transform the way you perceive setbacks and challenges. Instead of viewing obstacles as insurmountable roadblocks, a growth mindset encourages you to see them as opportunities for learning and development. Embracing change, rather than fearing it, allows you to continuously improve and adapt. This mindset is particularly useful in health journeys, where progress is rarely linear. By accepting that setbacks are part of the process, you can maintain resilience and keep moving forward. This adaptability not only enhances your health outcomes but also builds a stronger, more resilient mindset that extends into other areas of life.

Setting intentions for ongoing growth is a powerful way to align your actions with your evolving health goals. Intentions act as a north star, guiding you toward the areas you wish to develop further. They help you identify new opportunities for exploration, whether it's trying a different dietary approach, incorporating new physical activities, or learning more about the gut-brain connection. Committing to lifelong learning ensures that you're always open to new information and ideas. This openness fosters a continual process of self-improvement, allowing you to refine your approach as you gain more knowledge and experience. By setting clear intentions, you create a purposeful path forward, one that encourages growth and fulfillment.

As you reflect on these themes, consider how they fit into the larger picture of your health journey. Recognize that the insights gained from self-reflection, the resilience built through a growth mindset, and the clarity provided by setting intentions all contribute to a holistic approach to wellness. These elements work together to create a dynamic, evolving process that empowers you to take charge of your health. In the next chapter, we will explore how cultivating long-term health habits can reinforce these insights and lead to sustainable wellbeing.

11

CULTIVATING LONG-TERM HEALTH HABITS

T hink of your health journey as tending to a garden. Each small, consistent action you take—like watering or weeding—may not seem like much at the moment, but over time, these incremental efforts compound, yielding a lush and thriving garden. Your health is no different. Consistency is the gentle force that transforms sporadic efforts into lasting change, much like how a daily drop of water can wear away stone. When you commit to regular habits, you lay a foundation for long-term success, allowing small victories to build into significant progress.

Consistency plays a crucial role in reinforcing positive habits. Imagine each routine as a brick in a sturdy wall, each habit supporting the next, creating a structure that withstands the test of time. Establishing a routine makes health-related activities a non-negotiable part of your daily life.

These habits become second nature, much like brushing your teeth or locking the door when you leave home. When healthy choices are woven into the fabric of your everyday life, they require less conscious effort, freeing your mind for other pursuits. This compounding effect is the secret to achieving your health goals, turning ambitious dreams into attainable realities.

The power of consistency lies not just in its physical benefits but also in its psychological impact. Regular habits boost confidence by providing a sense of accomplishment, like crossing tasks off a checklist. Each completed task fuels motivation, creating a positive feedback loop that propels you forward. Consistency also reduces decision fatigue, the mental exhaustion that comes from making too many choices. When habits are ingrained, they require less mental energy, freeing you from the constant burden of decision-making. This mental clarity allows you to focus on more creative or challenging endeavors, enhancing your overall quality of life.

To maintain consistency, consider integrating simple strategies into your routine. Start by setting reminders for daily health activities, using your phone or a planner to keep you on track. These gentle nudges act as supportive guides, helping you stay committed to your goals. Additionally, habit-tracking apps can be valuable tools in monitoring progress. They provide visual representations of your achievements, offering encouragement and accountability.

Seeing your progress displayed in graphs or charts can be incredibly motivating, reinforcing the importance of each small step you take.

Practical examples of consistent health practices include simple routines that make a big difference over time. Begin your day by drinking a glass of water, hydrating your body and kickstarting your metabolism. This small act, when repeated daily, can have a cumulative effect on your overall health. Another practice is maintaining a gratitude journal. Taking a few moments each day to jot down things you're thankful for can shift your mindset, fostering positivity and reducing stress. These practices, though small, create ripples of change, contributing to your long-term health journey.

Interactive Element: Habit-Building Checklist

- Choose one new health habit to focus on this week.
- Set a specific time each day to practice this habit.
- Use a habit-tracking app or journal to record your progress.
- Reflect on how the habit impacts your day and adjust as needed.
- Celebrate each day you successfully practice your habit.

By weaving consistency into your daily routine, you create a sturdy foundation for health, much like a gardener who diligently tends to their plants. Over time, these efforts will bear fruit, leading to a life rich in vitality and fulfillment.

11.1 OVERCOMING SETBACKS: STAYING ON TRACK

Setbacks are as much a part of life as the air we breathe. They are the unexpected twists in our health journey that challenge our resolve and test our resilience. It's easy to feel discouraged when things don't go as planned, but it's important to remember that setbacks are not failures; they are merely detours on the path to success. Everyone faces them, and acknowledging their inevitability can help normalize the experience. By viewing setbacks as temporary and surmountable, you can shift your perspective from defeat to opportunity. This mindset encourages resilience, allowing you to bounce back stronger and more determined than before.

When setbacks occur, it's crucial to have strategies in place to help you regain momentum. Start by reassessing your goals. Sometimes a setback is a sign that your goals need tweaking. Are they realistic? Do they align with your current lifestyle and resources? Adjusting your goals to better fit your circumstances can reinvigorate your commitment and make the path forward more manageable. Additionally, seek support from a mentor or community. Sharing your experiences with others who understand can provide the encouragement and accountability you need to get back on track. Whether it's a friend, family member, or support group, having someone to lean on can make all the difference in overcoming obstacles.

Maintaining a positive mindset is vital in the face of setbacks. It's easy to spiral into negative thinking, but practicing self-compassion and forgiveness can help you stay optimistic. Remind yourself that everyone makes mistakes and that it's okay to stumble. Celebrate small wins along the way to boost your morale. These victories, no matter how minor, serve as reminders of your progress and potential. They reinforce the belief that you are capable of achieving your health goals, even if the road is bumpy. By focusing on what you have accomplished, rather than what you haven't, you can cultivate a mindset that propels you forward.

Reflection plays a crucial role in overcoming setbacks. It offers an opportunity to learn and grow from your experiences, turning challenges into valuable lessons. Take the time to reflect on what went wrong and why. Were there external factors beyond your control? Did you encounter internal obstacles like self-doubt or procrastination? Identifying these elements can help you develop a plan to prevent similar setbacks in the future. Perhaps you need to build in more flexibility or introduce new strategies to cope with stress. Whatever the case, reflection can illuminate the path forward, enabling you to approach your health goals with renewed clarity and purpose.

Reflection Section: Learning from Setbacks

Take a moment to think about a recent setback you've experienced. What did you learn from it? How did it make you feel, and how can you use this experience to inform your future actions? Write down your thoughts and consider what changes you might make to avoid similar challenges in the future.

11.2 MOTIVATION AND MINDSET: BUILDING RESILIENCE

Imagine waking up each day, driven not by the promise of a reward or the fear of punishment, but by a genuine sense of purpose and joy. This is the essence of intrinsic motivation— a force rooted in personal satisfaction and enjoyment. It's what makes you choose a salad not because you have to, but because you genuinely want to nourish your body. Aligning your health goals with your personal values taps into this intrinsic drive, making the process of change not just bearable but enjoyable. When your actions resonate with your core beliefs, they become more sustainable over time. You begin to find joy in the process itself, in the simple act of choosing what feels right for you. This internal motivation is like a wellspring of energy, fueling your journey with a sense of fulfillment and contentment that external rewards simply can't match.

To cultivate and maintain this motivation, consider visualizing your goals. Creating a vision board can be an inspiring way to keep your aspirations in sight. Gather images and words that reflect your health ambitions and arrange them on a board where you can see them daily. This visual reminder serves as a beacon, guiding you towards your desired outcomes and keeping your motivation alive. Alongside this, setting short-term milestones can provide immediate rewards and satisfaction. These smaller goals act like stepping stones, each one a tangible achievement that keeps you moving forward. Whether it's trying a new recipe or completing a week of regular exercise, these victories build momentum, reinforcing your commitment to your broader health objectives.

A growth mindset complements this motivation by encouraging resilience and adaptability. When you view challenges as opportunities for development, you transform obstacles into stepping stones. Instead of shying away from difficulties, you embrace them as essential parts of the learning process. This mindset turns effort into a path to mastery, where each attempt, whether successful or not, brings you closer to your goal. By focusing on the process rather than the outcome, you cultivate a sense of resilience that permeates all aspects of your life. This resilient mindset allows you to adapt and thrive, even in the face of adversity.

Changing perspectives can significantly enhance resilience. Consider reframing failures as learning experiences. When you stumble, view it as a chance to gain insight and grow rather than a setback. This shift in perspective can turn disappointment into determination, motivating you to try again with renewed vigor. Additionally, focusing on progress rather than perfection can alleviate pressure and stress. Perfection is often an unattainable standard, but progress is always within reach. Celebrate the small steps forward, recognizing that each one is a testament to your persistence and dedication. This focus on progress helps maintain momentum, ensuring that you continue to move forward, even if the path isn't always smooth or straight.

Visual Element: Vision Board Inspiration

Create a vision board to visualize your health goals. Include images, words, and symbols that resonate with your aspirations. Place it in a space where you'll see it often, and use it as a source of daily inspiration and motivation.

11.3 THE RIPPLE EFFECT: IMPACTING FUTURE GENERATIONS

Your personal health habits extend beyond your own wellbeing. They ripple outwards, influencing your family and community in ways you might not immediately see. When children watch you make healthy choices, they learn by example. Imagine a child observing their parent choosing a balanced meal over fast food or taking a moment to meditate instead of reaching for a phone. These seemingly small actions plant seeds in young minds, teaching them about self-care and wellness. This modeling of behavior is powerful. It shapes the attitudes and habits of future generations, setting them on a path to healthier lives.

Sharing your knowledge and resources with peers is another way to extend the positive effects of your health journey. When you discuss the benefits of a new exercise routine or share a healthy recipe, you open the door for others to explore their own health. This exchange of ideas and experiences fosters a community of wellness, where individuals support and inspire one another. It's a collective effort that can lead to broader health improvements within your social circle. By being open about your health journey, you encourage others to embark on their own, amplifying the impact of your choices.

Education is a cornerstone for creating lasting change. By teaching children about nutrition and self-care from a young age, you empower them with the knowledge to make informed decisions. Schools play a crucial role in this educational process. Encouraging open discussions about health in the classroom can demystify wellness and make it more approachable. It's about equipping the next generation with the tools they need to prioritize their health. When children understand the why and how of maintaining their wellbeing, they are more likely to adopt these practices into adulthood, creating a healthier society.

Community initiatives are vital for collective health improvement. Imagine local wellness events or workshops that bring people together to learn about nutrition, fitness, and mental health. These gatherings can foster a sense of community, where individuals feel supported in their health pursuits. Community programs can also advocate for policies that enhance public health, such as improved access to nutritious food or safe spaces for physical activity. By participating in or organizing these initiatives, you contribute to a culture of health that benefits everyone, creating an environment where wellness is prioritized and celebrated.

Personal health choices can leave a lasting legacy. Establishing family traditions centered around health, such as cooking healthy meals together or going for regular family walks, creates memories and instills values that persist through generations. These traditions become part of your family's identity, influencing the choices of your children and their children. Additionally, creating educational materials or guides based on your health experiences can serve as a resource for others. Whether it's a blog, a booklet, or a simple list of tips, sharing your insights helps others navigate their own health journeys.

In this way, your personal health habits are not just about you. They are a contribution to the world around you, influencing those you love and the communities you are part of. Your choices today can shape the future, creating a ripple effect that extends far beyond your immediate reach. The next chapter will delve deeper into how we can continue to nurture our wellbeing, exploring the comprehensive strategies that support a lifetime of health.

12

ENVISIONING A HARMONIOUS LIFE

I magine waking up each morning not feeling the weight of fatigue pulling you back into the sheets, but rather, a buoyant energy urging you to seize the day. Your skin, once a reflection of stress and imbalance, now glows with vitality, a testament to the harmony within. This is not a dream; it's the reality of balanced gut health—a reality within your reach. A well-functioning gut doesn't just make digestion smoother; it transforms your entire being. With enhanced energy levels, you'll notice a spring in your step as you tackle daily tasks with newfound vigor. This vitality stems from the gut's crucial role in nutrient absorption, ensuring your body gets the fuel it needs to thrive. Moreover, a healthy gut reduces gastrointestinal discomfort, freeing you from the shackles of bloating and irregularity.

Beyond the physical, the benefits of gut health extend to your mental and emotional realms. Have you ever experienced a foggy mind, struggling to focus on even the simplest tasks? A balanced gut can be your ally in clearing that haze. By supporting the production of neurotransmitters like serotonin, your gut aids in sharpening mental clarity and focus. This clarity isn't just about acing that math test or delivering a stellar presentation; it's about feeling present and engaged in everyday life. Additionally, as your gut nurtures emotional stability, you'll find yourself more resilient in the face of stress. Anxiety, often an unwelcome companion, diminishes as you build emotional resilience. This newfound stability allows you to navigate challenges with a calm confidence, transforming how you interact with the world around you.

As your physical and emotional health flourishes, the ripple effects extend into your social life. Picture yourself at a social gathering, feeling assured and at ease, engaging in lively conversations without the nagging distraction of discomfort. Improved gut health boosts your confidence, allowing you to connect with others more authentically. This connection is not just about being the life of the party; it's about fostering deeper relationships through enhanced communication and empathy. When you feel good, it's easier to be present for others, to listen and respond with genuine understanding. This empathy enriches your interactions, creating a supportive social network that uplifts both you and those around you.

Consider the story of Mia, a young woman who battled chronic fatigue for years. No matter how much she slept, she never felt rested. It wasn't until she focused on improving her gut health through a diverse, plant-based diet that she experienced a dramatic shift. Her energy levels soared, and she found herself participating in activities she once thought impossible. Similarly, Jake, who struggled with mood swings, discovered the power of gut health in stabilizing his emotions. By incorporating probiotics and reducing sugar intake, Jake not only improved his mood but also strengthened his relationships. His newfound emotional balance allowed him to communicate more effectively, deepening his connections with friends and family.

Reflection Section: Visualizing Your Transformation

Take a moment to close your eyes and visualize the version of yourself that thrives with optimal gut health. Picture your daily routine filled with energy, clarity, and positive interactions. Reflect on the steps you can take to bring this vision to life. Consider journaling your thoughts and setting small, achievable goals to support your gut health journey. This reflection is not just about imagining a better future; it's about crafting a roadmap to make it your reality.

12.1 HARMONY IN LIFE: ACHIEVING BALANCE

Living a harmonious life is like conducting an orchestra where each section plays its part to create a symphony of wellbeing. It's about finding a rhythm that integrates your physical, mental, and emotional health seamlessly. Imagine having a day where your actions and values align, where what you do is a reflection of who you are at your core. This harmony enhances your overall wellbeing, allowing you to move through life with a sense of purpose and clarity. Balancing these aspects means listening to your body, nurturing your mind with positive thoughts, and fostering emotions that uplift rather than weigh you down. It's the subtle alignment between what you believe and how you act daily, creating a life that feels authentic and fulfilling.

Maintaining this balance amidst life's demands can be challenging, but practical strategies can help you achieve it. Start with time management techniques that prioritize what truly matters to you. Set aside time each day for activities that nourish your soul, whether it's reading, walking, or simply being still. Scheduling these moments can prevent the chaos of daily life from overwhelming you. Setting priorities that reflect your personal values is another key strategy. Identify what's most important to you and allocate your energy accordingly. Whether it's family, career, or personal growth, focusing on these priorities ensures that your actions are aligned with your values.

Mindfulness plays a pivotal role in maintaining this harmony. By practicing mindfulness, you center yourself and cultivate awareness of the present moment. Daily mindfulness exercises, such as meditation or deep breathing, help ground you, reducing stress and enhancing emotional resilience. When you make decisions mindfully, you're more likely to choose options that align with your values and goals. This alignment fosters a sense of peace and satisfaction, reducing the internal conflict that can disrupt balance. Mindful decision-making involves pausing before reacting, considering your choices, and proceeding with intention. It's about making choices that resonate with your inner self, promoting harmony in your life.

Your path to harmony is uniquely yours, and it's essential to personalize it to reflect your desires and aspirations. Consider creating a vision board that visually represents your personal goals. Collect images and words that inspire you, and arrange them in a way that motivates you daily. This board serves as a tangible reminder of what you're working towards, keeping your goals at the forefront of your mind. Journaling is another powerful tool for reflection and progress tracking. By regularly noting your experiences, you can identify patterns, celebrate successes, and make adjustments as needed. This practice encourages self-awareness and growth, helping you stay aligned with your vision of a harmonious life.

12.2 SUSTAINABLE PRACTICES FOR A BETTER WORLD

Imagine a world where every small choice you make contributes to the health of the planet. This isn't just a dream; it's a reality within your grasp through sustainable living. Your everyday actions, like reducing waste and choosing eco-friendly products, play a significant role in shaping a healthier environment. Consider the impact of mindful consumption. By being conscious of what you buy and how you dispose of it, you can significantly cut down on waste. Opt for products with minimal packaging, recycle whenever possible, and embrace a minimalist approach to purchasing. Instead of using disposable items, choose reusable alternatives like stainless steel water bottles and cloth shopping bags. These small changes reduce waste and conserve resources, making a positive impact on the planet.

The ripple effect of sustainable practices extends beyond personal health and into the community, fostering broader environmental and social change. By supporting local farmers, you not only enjoy fresher produce but also contribute to reducing the carbon footprint associated with transporting goods over long distances. This support helps sustain local economies and encourages sustainable farming practices, which are better for the soil and biodiversity. Participating in community clean-up initiatives is another way to contribute. These activities not only beautify your surroundings but also raise awareness about environmental issues, inspiring others to take action. They create a sense of community and shared responsibility, reinforcing the idea that individual actions can lead to substantial collective impact.

Incorporating sustainability into your daily routine doesn't require drastic changes; it involves thoughtful planning and conscious choices. Meal planning is an effective strategy to minimize food waste. By planning your meals, you can buy only what you need, reducing the likelihood of food spoiling before it's used. This approach not only saves money but also ensures that resources are used efficiently. When shopping, bring reusable bags and containers to reduce reliance on single-use plastics. These simple steps can significantly reduce your environmental footprint, making your lifestyle more sustainable. Choosing eco-friendly products for personal care, like biodegradable toothbrushes and natural skincare, further aligns your daily habits with sustainability goals.

Education is a powerful tool in promoting sustainable practices, and you have the ability to share knowledge within your community. Hosting educational workshops or discussions about sustainability can open dialogues and spread awareness about its benefits. These workshops provide a platform for exchanging ideas, experiences, and solutions for living more sustainably. Sharing resources and tips with friends and family can inspire them to adopt sustainable habits, creating a ripple effect that extends beyond your immediate circle. This sharing of knowledge encourages others to make informed choices, amplifying the positive impact on the environment.

Interactive Element: Sustainable Living Checklist

Consider creating a checklist of sustainable actions tailored to your lifestyle. Include tasks like reducing energy consumption, composting waste, and supporting local businesses. Use this checklist to track your progress and reflect on how each action contributes to a healthier planet. Regularly review and update your checklist, adding new sustainable practices as you learn and grow. This simple tool not only keeps you accountable but also serves as a reminder of the positive changes you're making. It's a personal roadmap to sustainability, empowering you to make a difference every day.

12.3 THE FUTURE OF GUT HEALTH: A HOPEFUL OUTLOOK

Picture a world where your gut health is as personalized as your morning coffee order. Advances in gut health research are paving the way for a future where nutrition is tailored to your unique microbiome. Imagine being able to take a simple test that reveals the composition of your gut bacteria, allowing you to receive dietary recommendations tailored to enhance your personal health. This is the promise of personalized nutrition, driven by cutting-edge microbiome analysis. Such innovations are not just dreams of the future; they are becoming tangible realities, offering a bespoke approach to nutrition that considers your gut's distinct ecosystem. Alongside these advancements, the development of new probiotic and prebiotic formulations holds potential to revolutionize how we support gut health. By creating targeted supplements, researchers are working to ensure that your microbiome receives the exact strains of beneficial bacteria it needs to thrive.

Technology is rapidly transforming the landscape of gut health management, offering tools that empower you to take control of your digestive wellbeing. Mobile applications now allow you to track your dietary habits, monitor symptoms, and even connect with nutrition experts. These apps are like having a gut health coach in your pocket, guiding you towards better choices and helping you understand how different foods impact your body. Wearable devices, too, are entering the fray, designed to monitor digestive function in real time. Imagine a device that alerts you when your gut is under stress or when it's time to adjust your diet. These innovations make it easier than ever to be proactive about your gut health, providing insights that were once the domain of medical professionals.

As awareness of the gut's vital role in overall health continues to grow, we can envision a societal shift where gut health becomes a central focus in public health initiatives. Increased accessibility to gut health education means that more people will understand the importance of a balanced microbiome. Schools may integrate gut health into their health curriculums, teaching students from a young age about the impact of diet and lifestyle on their digestive system. Workplace wellness programs might emphasize gut health, offering resources and support to help employees make gut-friendly choices. These programs could include workshops on nutrition, stress management, and even workplace snacks that promote a healthy microbiome. Such initiatives would not only improve individual health but also enhance productivity and wellbeing on a larger scale.

Imagine a world where communities embrace gut health principles, creating environments that foster collective wellbeing. In this vision, neighborhood gardens are cultivated with diversity in mind, offering a range of produce that supports a healthy microbiome. Farmers' markets flourish, providing access to fresh, gut-friendly foods. Local gyms and wellness centers host classes and workshops focused on gut health, from yoga sessions designed to aid digestion to seminars on the gut-brain connection. These communities become hubs of health education and support, demonstrating the power of collective action in achieving wellness goals. As more people prioritize their gut health, the ripple effects could address pressing global health challenges, such as obesity and mental health disorders.

Visual Element: Future of Gut Health Infographic

Consider examining an infographic that outlines the emerging trends in gut health research and technology. This visual representation can provide a snapshot of what the future holds, from personalized nutrition to advanced wearable devices. Reviewing these developments can inspire you to explore new ways to support your gut health and stay informed about the latest advances. Keep this infographic as a reminder of the exciting possibilities that lie ahead, motivating you to embrace these innovations and integrate them into your life.

As we look toward the future, the role of gut health in achieving a healthier society becomes ever more promising. With continued research and a growing understanding of the microbiome, we are poised to unlock new levels of health and vitality.

CONCLUSION

As we come to the end of our journey together, I want to take a moment to reflect on the incredible insights we've uncovered about gut health and its far-reaching impact on our lives. Throughout this book, we've explored the intricate connections between the gut, emotional wellbeing, and the choices we make every day. We've seen how a holistic approach, one that embraces nutrition, mindfulness, and sustainable living, can transform our health and our world.

At the heart of this journey lies the gut, a complex and powerful system that influences every aspect of our wellbeing. Recent research has only begun to unravel the mysteries of the gut, revealing its crucial role in immunity, emotional balance, and vitality. The evidence is clear: when we nurture our gut health, we unlock a new level of wellness that radiates through our entire being.

Each chapter of this book has provided essential lessons and practical strategies to help you cultivate a thriving gut. From the benefits of a plant-based diet to the importance of stress management, from the power of probiotics to the value of consistency, these insights form a roadmap to better health. By incorporating these principles into your daily life, you can experience the transformative effects firsthand.

But knowledge alone is not enough. True change begins with reflection and action. I encourage you to take a moment to consider your own health journey. What changes are you inspired to make? What goals feel most meaningful to you? Use the tools and exercises provided in this book to create a plan that resonates with your unique needs and aspirations. Remember, every small step you take is a step towards a healthier, more vibrant you.

As you embark on this path, I invite you to envision the life that awaits you. Picture yourself waking up each morning with boundless energy, your mind clear and focused. Imagine facing challenges with resilience and grace, your emotional wellbeing fortified by a balanced gut. This is the promise of gut health—a promise that is within your reach.

Remember, you are not alone on this journey. Seek out the support of loved ones, friends, and wellness communities. Surround yourself with people who uplift and inspire you, who share your commitment to health and growth. These connections will nourish you, providing encouragement and accountability as you navigate the path ahead.

As you nurture your own health, I urge you to consider the broader impact of your choices. By adopting sustainable practices, like reducing waste and supporting local food systems, you contribute to the health of our planet. Your individual actions ripple outwards, shaping a world that is kinder, greener, and more resilient. In caring for your gut, you care for the future—not just your own, but that of generations to come.

This book is just the beginning. Your journey of health and discovery continues beyond these pages. Stay curious, stay informed, and stay committed to your wellbeing. Embrace the power of lifelong learning, knowing that each new insight brings you closer to your healthiest, most vibrant self.

As we part ways, I leave you with a final thought. Your health is your most precious gift, a sacred trust that deserves your unwavering devotion. By nurturing your gut, you nurture your entire being—body, mind, and soul. You have the power to transform your life, to create a reality that is brimming with vitality and joy. Embrace this power, and let it guide you towards a future that shines with the radiance of true health.

Remember, your journey is unique, and your progress is something to celebrate. Every choice you make in support of your gut health is a testament to your strength, your wisdom, and your commitment to a life well-lived. As you continue on this path, know that I am here, cheering you on every step of the way. Together, we can create a world where health and harmony thrive, where every gut is cherished, and every life is lived to its fullest potential.

So go forth with confidence, armed with the knowledge and tools you need to cultivate a thriving gut and a joyful life. The journey ahead is filled with endless possibilities, and I can't wait to see where it takes you. Here's to your health, your happiness, and the incredible adventure that awaits.

With heartfelt gratitude and mutual commitment!

Elsa Rivers

REFERENCES

- *The Immune System and Microbiome - NCI* https://www.cancer.gov/research/areas/public-health/immune-system-microbiome
- *The Brain-Gut Connection* https://www.hopkinsmedicine.org/health/wellness-and-prevention/the-brain-gut-connection
- *Gut microbiota functions: metabolism of nutrients and other ...* https://pmc.ncbi.nlm.nih.gov/articles/PMC5847071/
- *Gut microbiome in 2023: current and emerging research ...* https://www.gutmicrobiotaforhealth.com/gut-microbiome-in-2023-current-and-emerging-research-trends/
- *Microbiota–gut–brain axis and its therapeutic applications ...* https://www.nature.com/articles/s41392-024-01743-1
- *Serotonin in the gut: Blessing or a curse* https://www.sciencedirect.com/science/article/abs/pii/S0300908418301652
- *Gut feelings: associations of emotions and ...* https://pubmed.ncbi.nlm.nih.gov/36942524/
- *Probiotics' Effects in the Treatment of Anxiety and Depression* https://pmc.ncbi.nlm.nih.gov/articles/PMC10893170/
- *Effect of Plant-Based Diets on Gut Microbiota: A Systematic ...* https://pmc.ncbi.nlm.nih.gov/articles/PMC10057430/
- *Probiotics and prebiotics: What you should know* https://www.mayoclinic.org/healthy-lifestyle/nutrition-and-healthy-eating/expert-answers/probiotics/faq-20058065
- *Ultra-processed foods and food additives in gut health and ...* https://www.nature.com/articles/s41575-024-00893-5
- *Promoting gut health through diet: tips from dietitians for ...* https://www.gutmicrobiotaforhealth.com/promoting-gut-health-through-diet-tips-from-dietitians-for-sustainable-health/
- *Gut-associated lymphoid tissue - Wikipedia* https://en.wikipedia.org/wiki/Gut-associated_lymphoid_tissue#:~:text=Gut%

2Dassociated%20lymphoid%20tissue%20(GALT,from%20invasion%20in%20the%20gut.

- *Regulation of short-chain fatty acids in the immune system* https://pmc.ncbi.nlm.nih.gov/articles/PMC10196242/
- *Psychosocial stress-induced intestinal permeability in healthy ...* https://pmc.ncbi.nlm.nih.gov/articles/PMC10569989/#:~:text=It%20should%20be%20noted%20that,dysfunction%20(Hall%20et%20al.%2C
- *Fermented-food diet increases microbiome diversity ...* https://med.stanford.edu/news/all-news/2021/07/fermented-food-diet-increases-microbiome-diversity-lowers-inflammation.html
- *Stress, depression, diet, and the gut microbiota* https://pmc.ncbi.nlm.nih.gov/articles/PMC7213601/#:~:text=Stress%20and%20depression%20can%20increase,19%E2%80%A2%E2%80%A2%2C20%5D.
- *Gut microbiome diversity is associated with sleep physiology ...* https://pmc.ncbi.nlm.nih.gov/articles/PMC6779243/#:~:text=We%20found%20that%20total%20microbiome,for%20its%20effects%20on%20sleep.
- *Exercise for digestion: Yoga, stretching, walking, breathing ...* https://www.medicalnewstoday.com/articles/exercises-to-help-digestion
- *Mindful Eating: A Review Of How The Stress-Digestion ...* https://pmc.ncbi.nlm.nih.gov/articles/PMC7219460/
- *Bloating Causes and Treatment - Digestive Disorders* https://www.webmd.com/digestive-disorders/remedies-for-bloating
- *Food allergy vs. food intolerance: What's the difference?* https://www.mayoclinic.org/diseases-conditions/food-allergy/expert-answers/food-allergy/faq-20058538
- *High-fiber foods - Nutrition and healthy eating* https://www.mayoclinic.org/healthy-lifestyle/nutrition-and-healthy-eating/in-depth/high-fiber-foods/art-20050948
- *Exploring the Influence of Gut Microbiome on Energy ...* https://pmc.ncbi.nlm.nih.gov/articles/PMC10334151/

- *Adolescence, the Microbiota-Gut-Brain Axis, and ...* https://www.sciencedirect.com/science/article/abs/pii/S0006322323016268
- *Stress, depression, diet, and the gut microbiota* https://pmc.ncbi.nlm.nih.gov/articles/PMC7213601/#:~:text=Psychological%20stress%20and%20depression%20can,%2C%20inflamma-tion%2C%20and%20autonomic%20alterations.
- *Hormones and Gastrointestinal Problems: Link & Symptoms* https://www.verywellhealth.com/hormones-and-gastrointestinal-problems-5216476
- *Nutrient absorption and intestinal adaptation with ageing* https://pubmed.ncbi.nlm.nih.gov/11977925/
- *How to Communicate Health Updates with Friends & Family* https://www.palhelps.com/library/keeping-loved-ones-in-the-loop-how-to-communicate-health-updates-with-friends-family/
- *Weight Stigma and Food Bias* https://emilyprogram.com/blog/weight-stigma-and-food-bias/
- *Developing Your Support System - UB School of Social Work* https://socialwork.buffalo.edu/resources/self-care-starter-kit/additional-self-care-resources/developing-your-support-system.html
- *The Digital Shift in Wellness Programs | Cape Fox FCG* https://capefoxfcg.com/mediacenter/leveraging-technology-in-health-promotion-the-digital-shift-in-wellness-programs/
- *The Microbiota–Gut–Brain Axis: Psychoneuroimmunological ...* https://pmc.ncbi.nlm.nih.gov/articles/PMC10059722/#:~:text=According%20to%20recent%20studies%2C%20the,and%20Oscil-libacter%20increase%20gene%20expression
- *The open secret to digestive health* https://theayurvedicclinic.com/the-open-secret-to-digestive-health/
- *Deep meditation may alter gut microbes for better health* https://bmjgroup.com/deep-meditation-may-alter-gut-microbes-for-better-health/#:~:text=Regular%20deep%20meditation%2C%20practised%20for,open%20access%20jour-nal%20General%20Psychiatry.

- *Precision Nutrition Unveiled: Gene–Nutrient Interactions ...* https:// pmc.ncbi.nlm.nih.gov/articles/PMC10935146/
- *Best Gut Health Apps of 2020* https://www.healthline.com/health/ digestive-health/top-iphone-android-apps-gut-health
- *Transformation stories | The Gut Health Doctor* https://www. theguthealthdoctor.com/transformation-stories#:~:text=After% 20being%20diagnosed% 20with%20an,and%20overall%20health%20have%20improved.
- *Gut Microbiota Associated With Effectiveness And ...* https://pmc.ncbi. nlm.nih.gov/articles/PMC8908961/
- *Setting SMART Goals to Improve Your Health* https:// northcitydiagnostic.com/setting-smart-goals-to-improve-your- health/
- *The Power of Consistency: Achieving Your Health Goals ...* https:// mdmonthly.com/the-power-of-consistency-achieving-your- health-goals-throughout-the-year/
- *The Health Benefits of Resilience—And How to Cultivate ...* https:// www.psychologytoday.com/us/blog/the-healing-factor/202405/ the-health-benefits-of-resilience-and-how-to-cultivate-more-of- it
- *Intrinsic Motivation Theory: Overview, Factors, and Examples* https:// www.healthline.com/health/intrinsic-motivation
- *The Impact of Personal Decisions on the Health ...* https://www.nphic. org/news/featured-topics/1295-personal-health-is-public- health-the-impact-of-personal-decisions-on-the-health-of-the- community
- *The Role of Gut Microbiota in Anxiety, Depression, and Other ...* https://pmc.ncbi.nlm.nih.gov/articles/PMC10384867/#:~:text= Several%20gut%20microbiota%2C%20especially% 20Firmicutes,depression%2C%20and%20other%20mental%20disorders.
- *Effect of Plant-Based Diets on Gut Microbiota: A Systematic ...* https:// pmc.ncbi.nlm.nih.gov/articles/PMC10057430/
- *The Microbiome Connecting Thread: From Farm to Food to ...* https://

sustainability.illinois.edu/the-microbiome-connection-from-farm-to-food-to-human-health/

- *Gut microbiome in 2023: current and emerging research ...* https://www.gutmicrobiotaforhealth.com/gut-microbiome-in-2023-current-and-emerging-research-trends/